The Great Seated Stretch Tubing Book

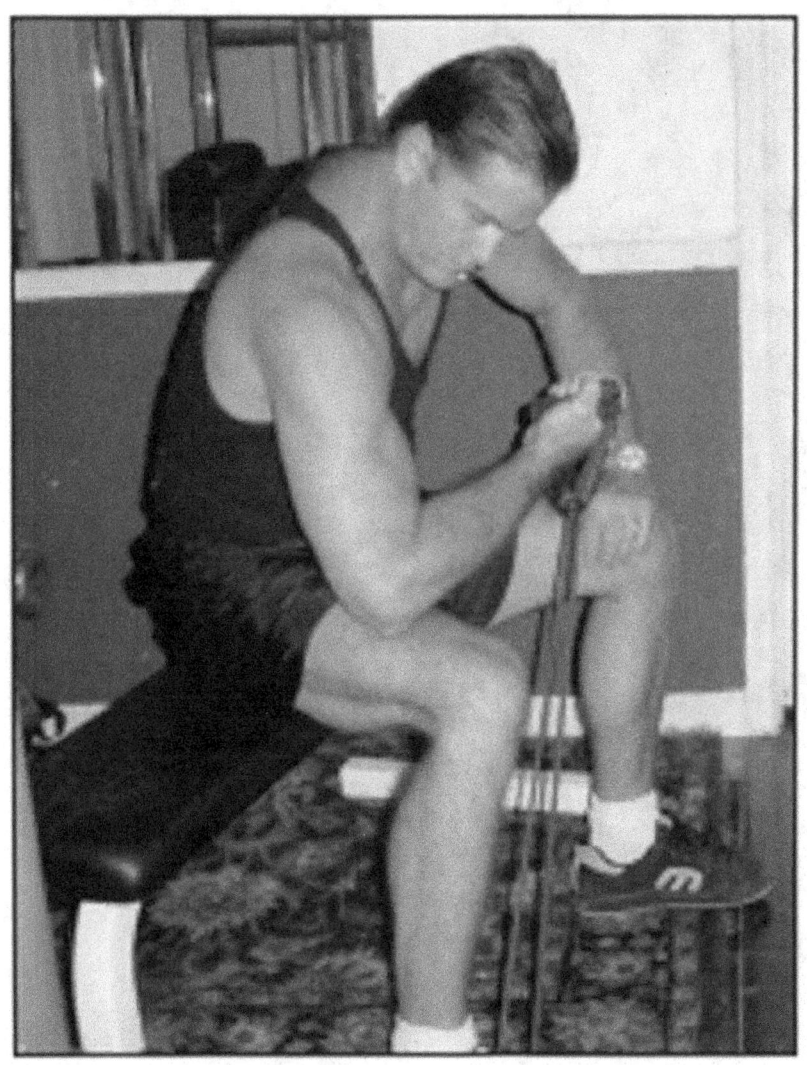

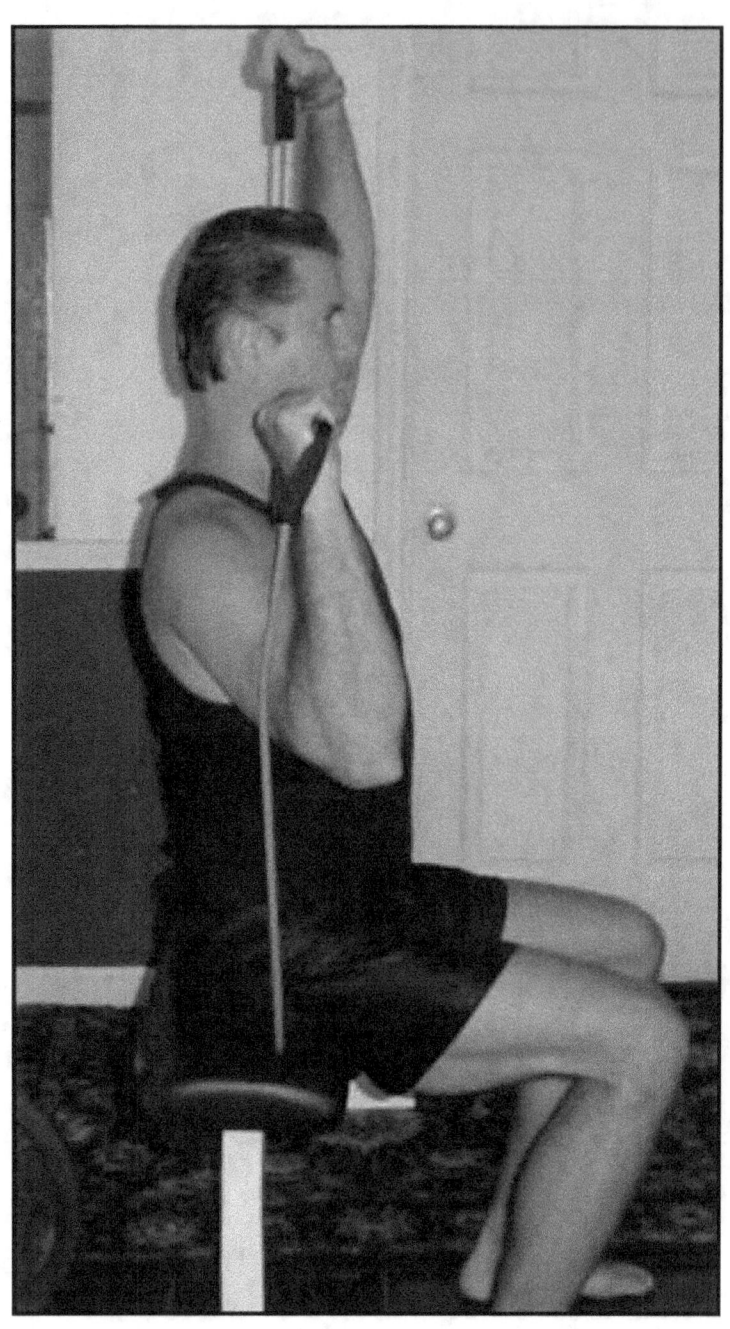

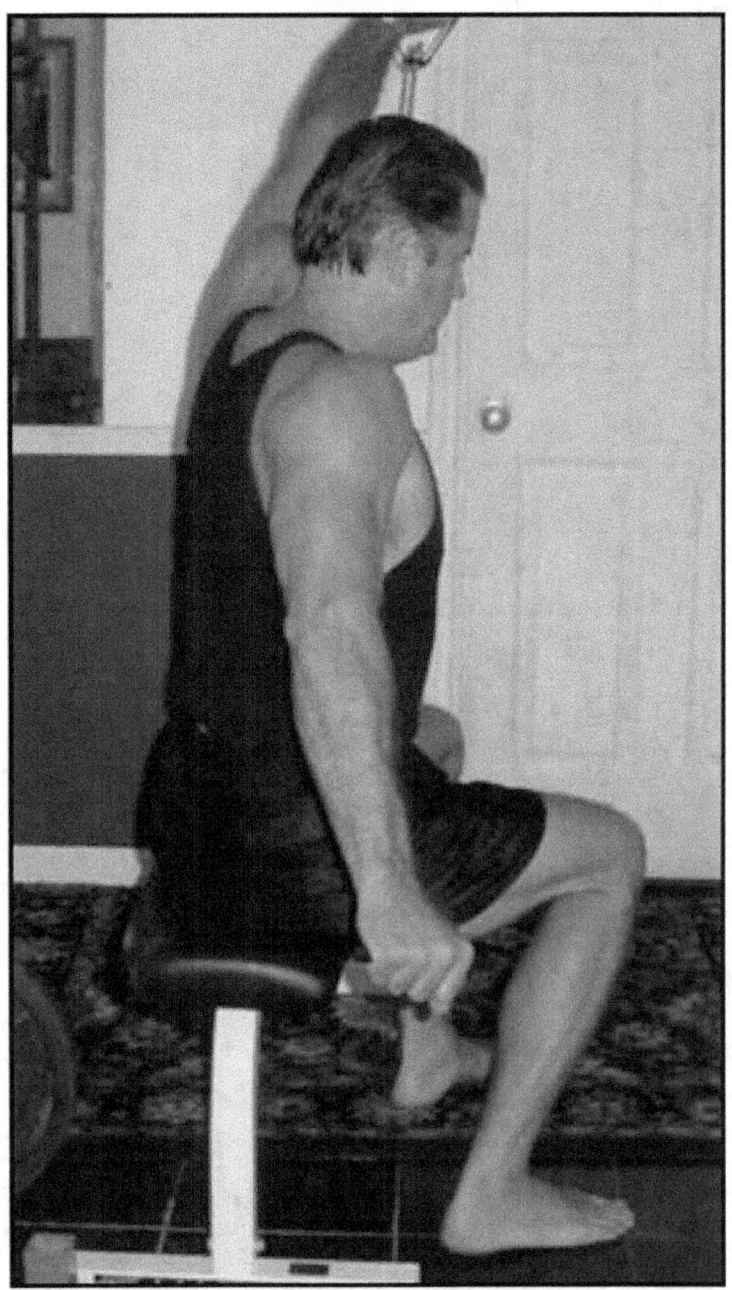

Here we are sitting and we extended one arm up and to the side and one arm back.

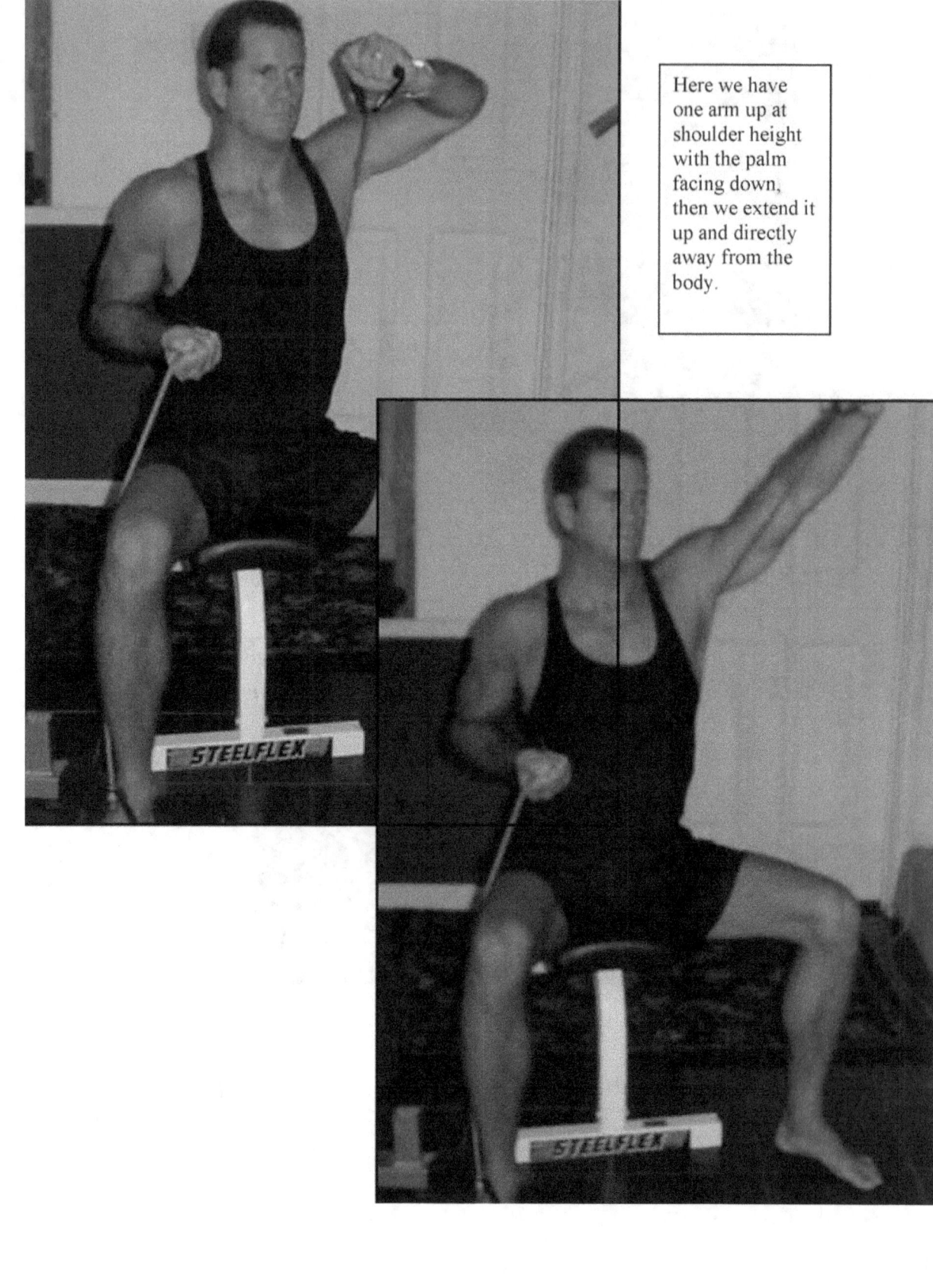

Here we have one arm up at shoulder height with the palm facing down, then we extend it up and directly away from the body.

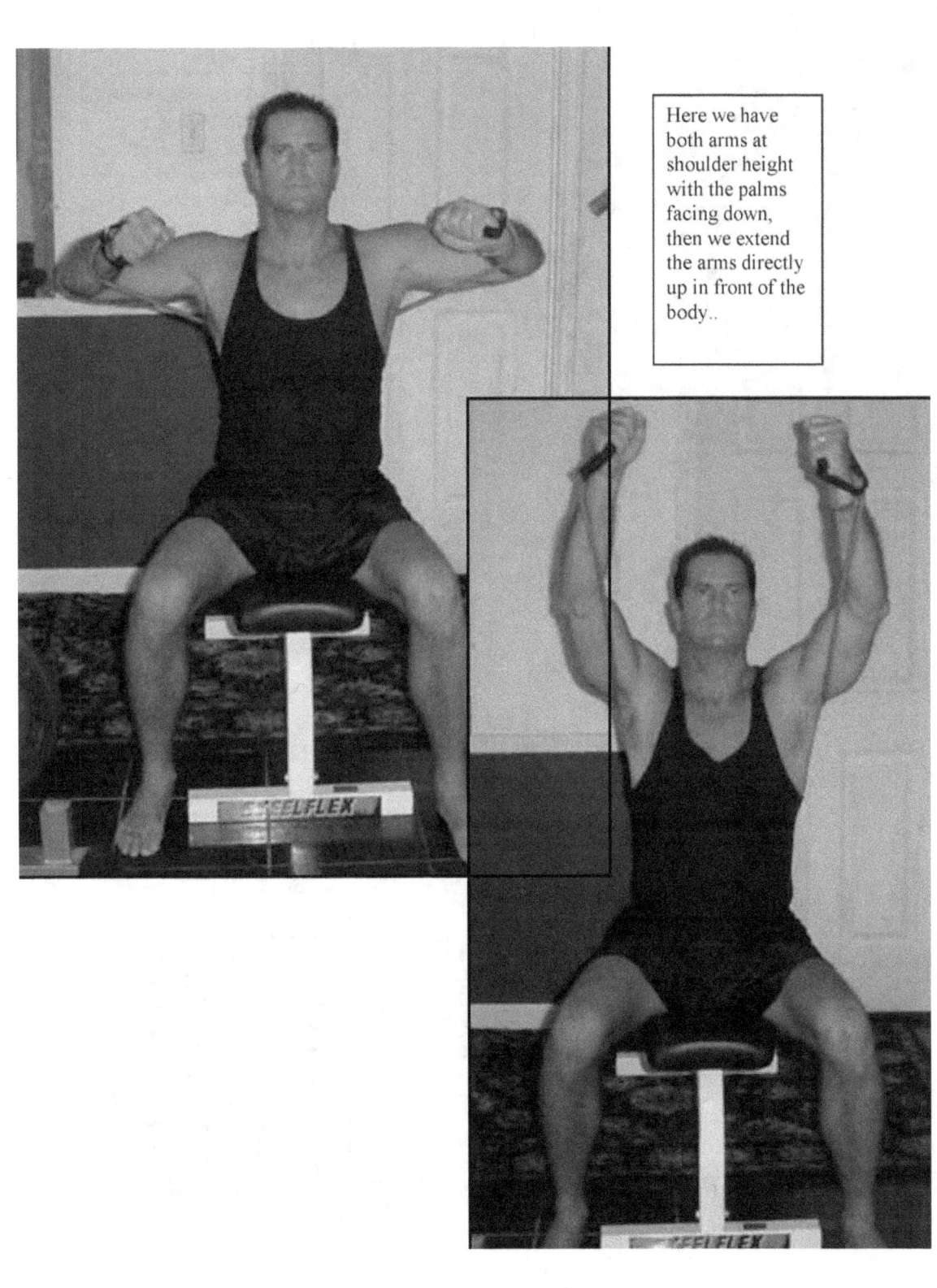

Here we have both arms at shoulder height with the palms facing down, then we extend the arms directly up in front of the body..

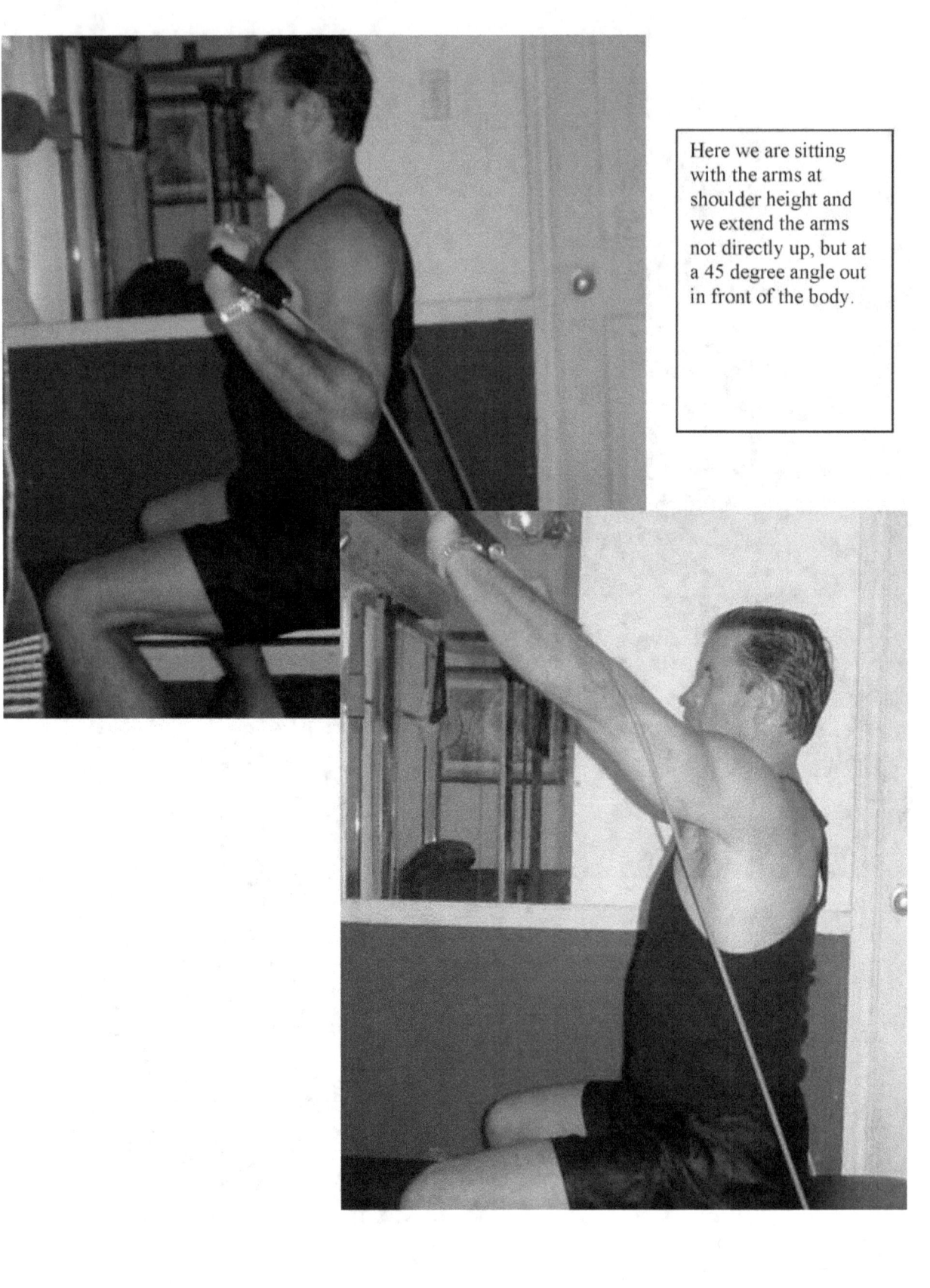

Here we are sitting with the arms at shoulder height and we extend the arms not directly up, but at a 45 degree angle out in front of the body.

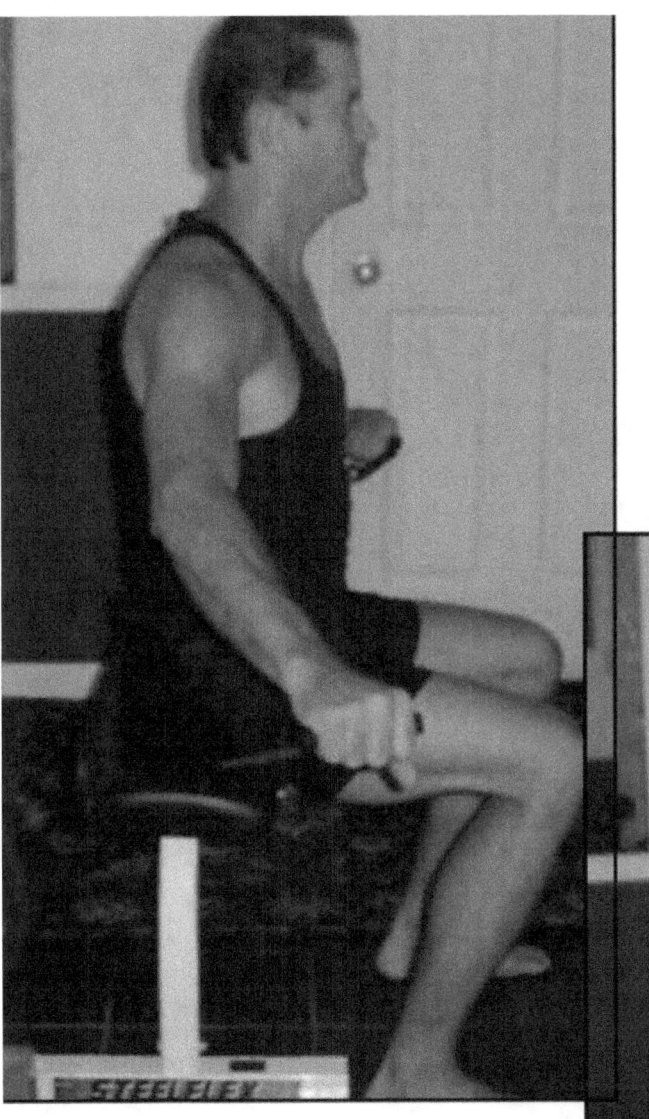

Here we are sitting
with the arms already
out to the sides and
then we extend the
arms up all the way up
and to the side.

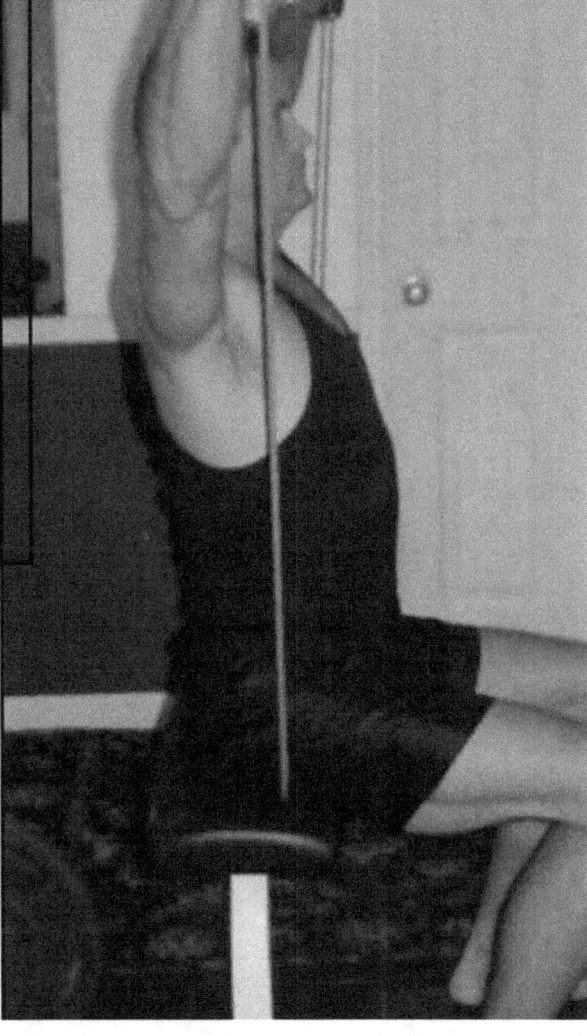

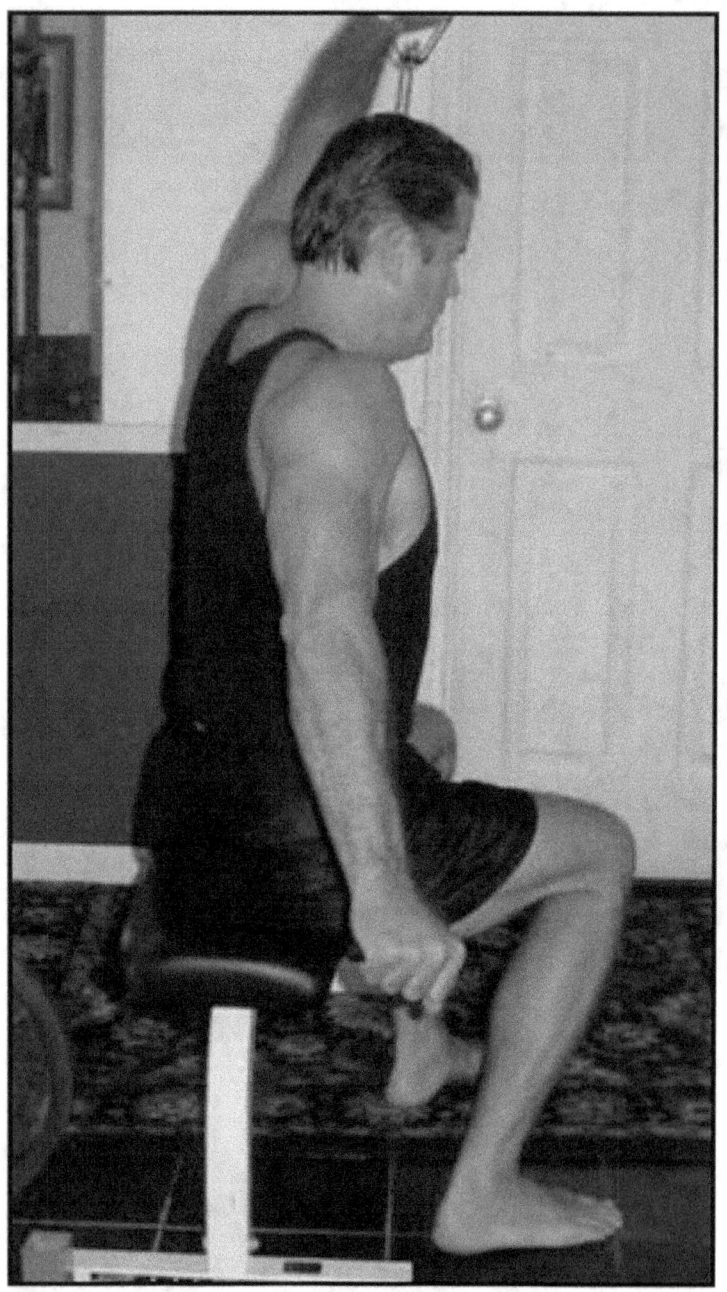

This is a variation with one arm going up and one arm going back. .

Here are lying down with the leg holding the tube and the arms up, then we pull the arms back across the body fully to the sides.

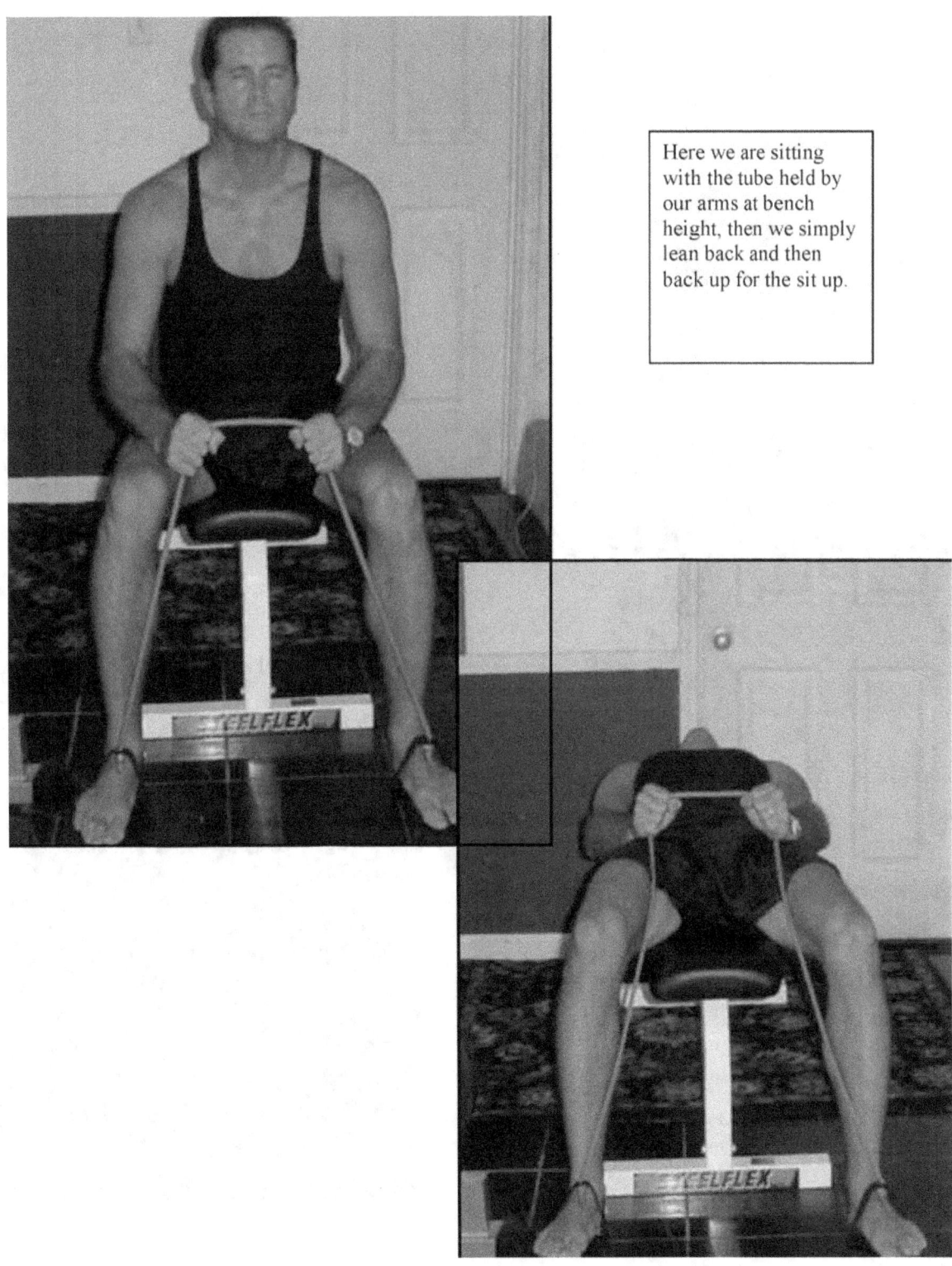

Here we are sitting with the tube held by our arms at bench height, then we simply lean back and then back up for the sit up.

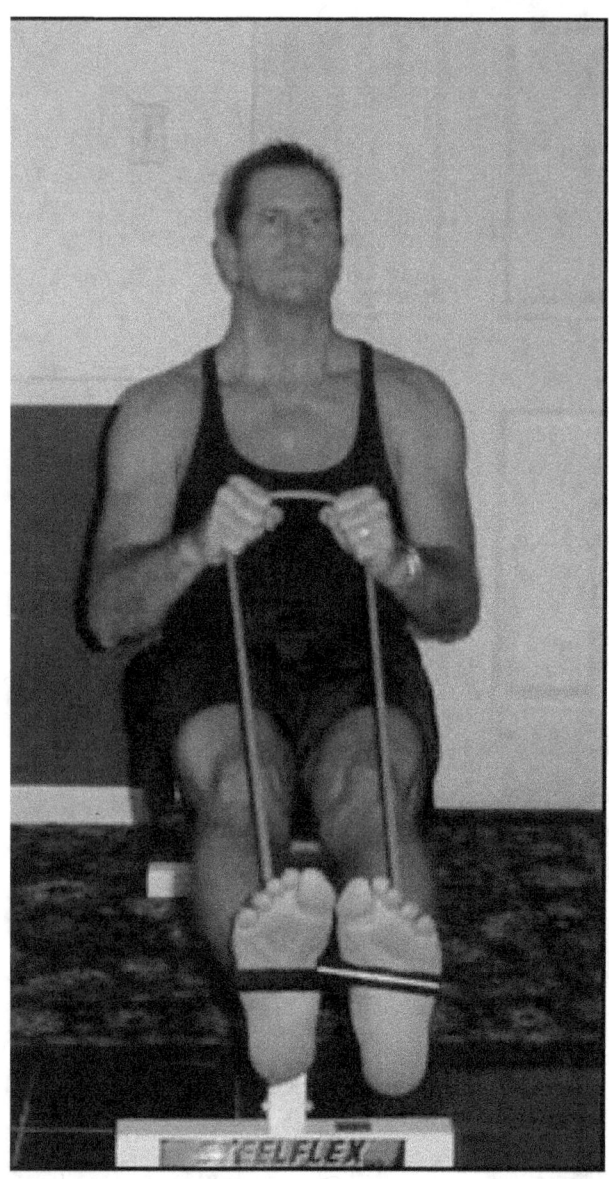

Here we are sitting with the tube held by our arms and around the feet, the feet are extended in front of the body, then we do our sit ups.

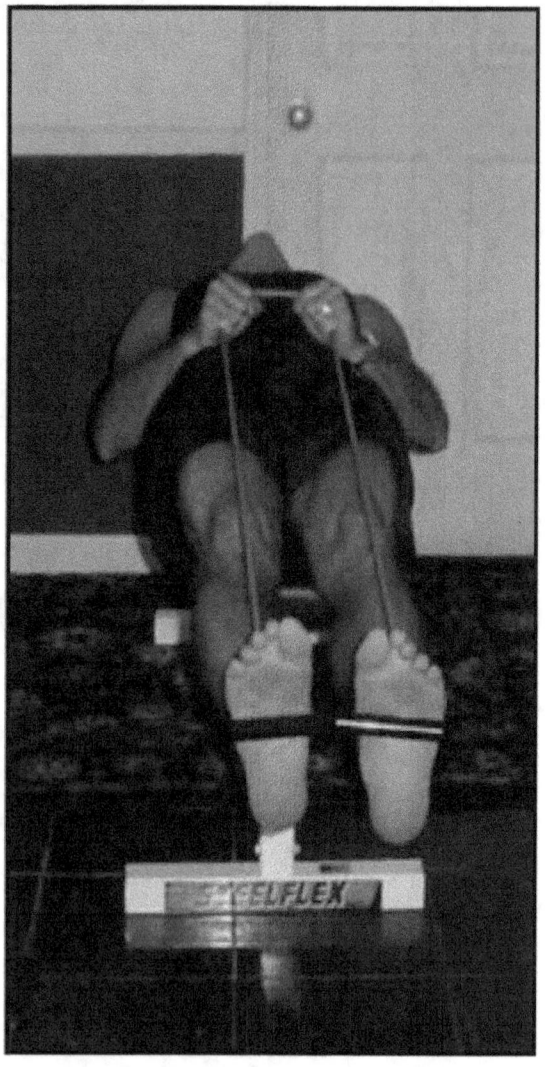

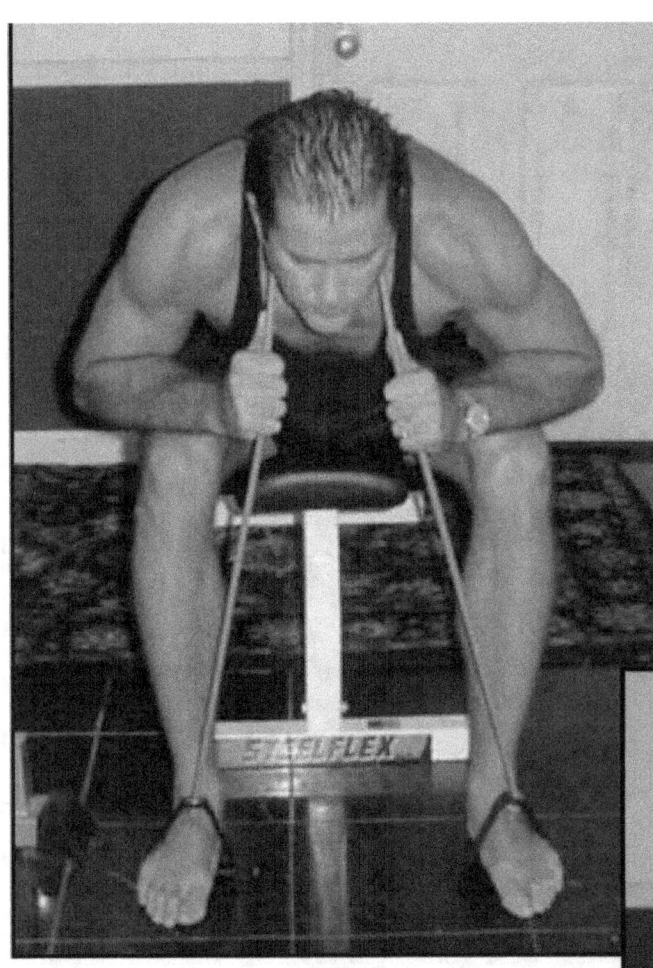

Here we are sitting with the tube held by our arms around the neck, while we are bent forward, then we sit up.

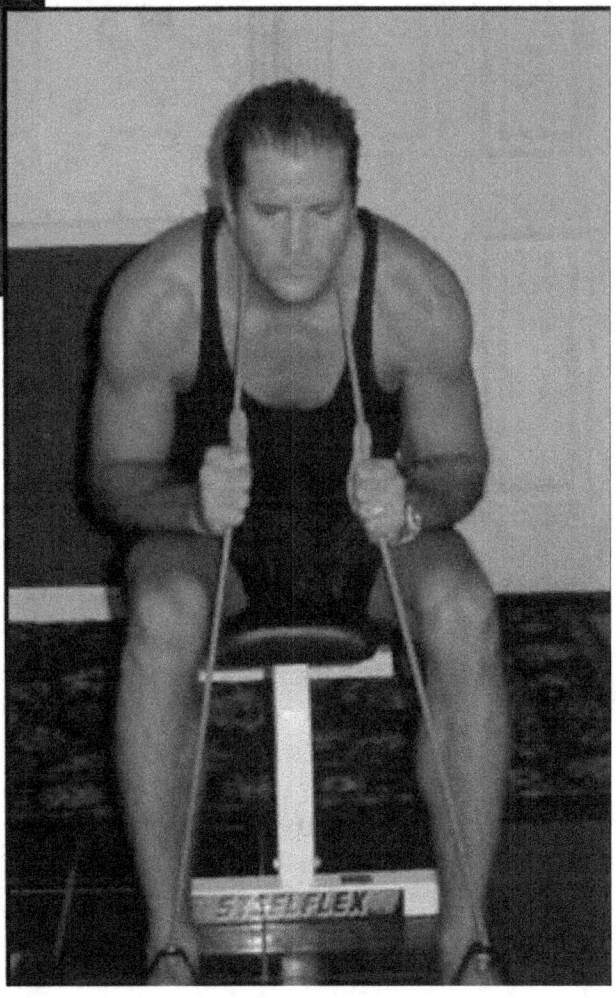

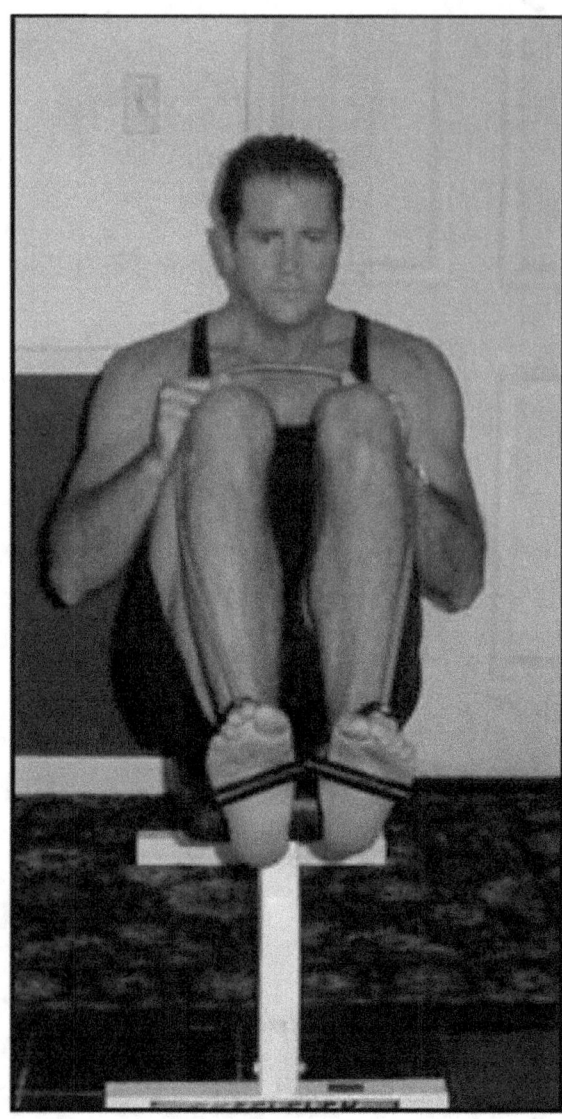

Here we work the lower abs by holding the tube with our feet, keeping or legs pulled in to the body, then extended out for the move. .

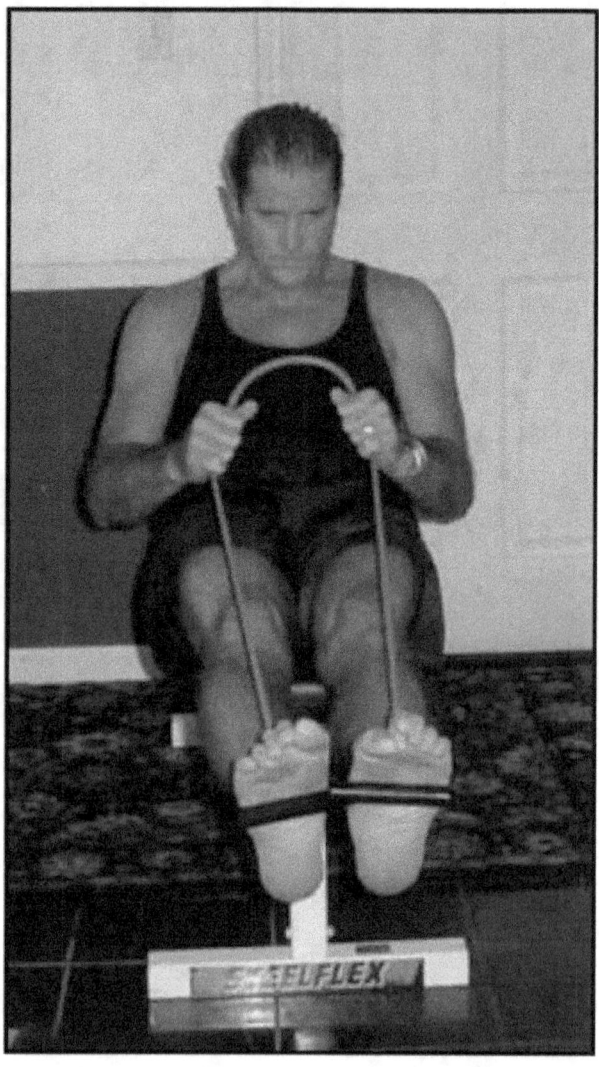

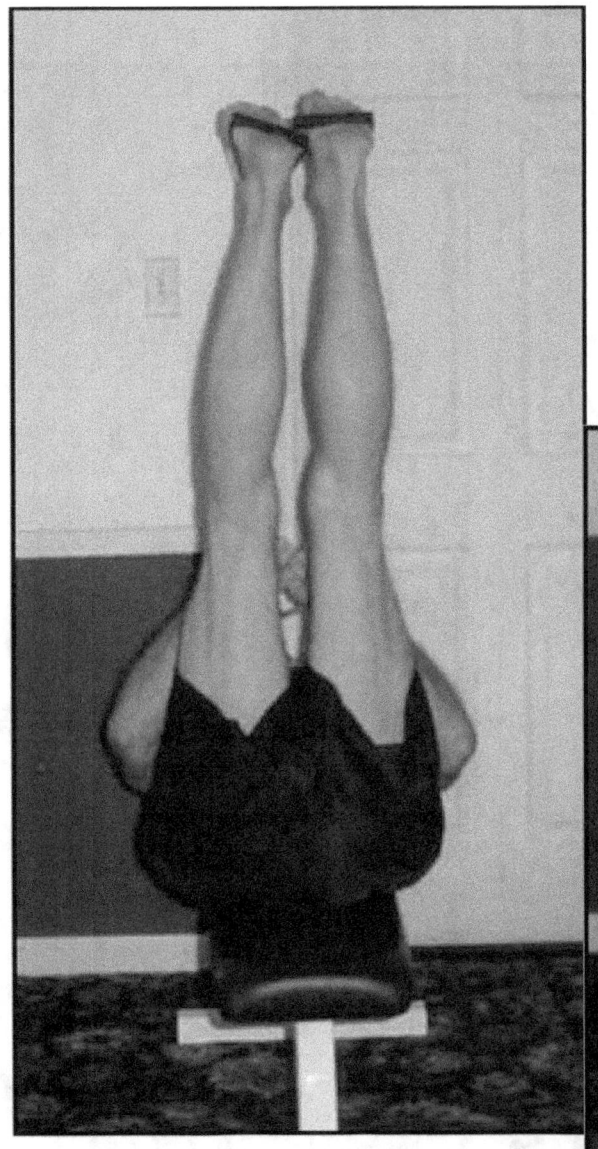

This a leg lift using the tube held by our feet. Simply lift the legs up and then down. .

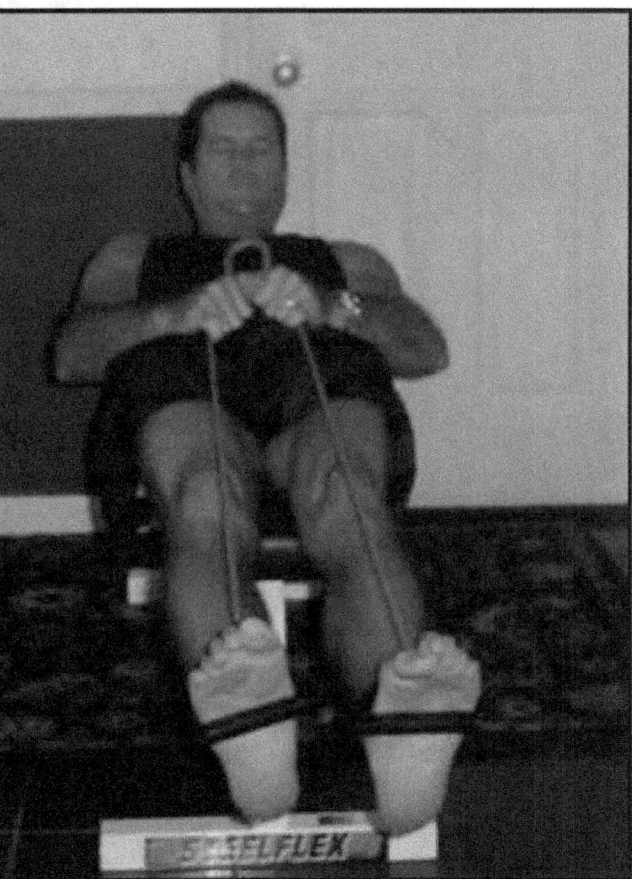

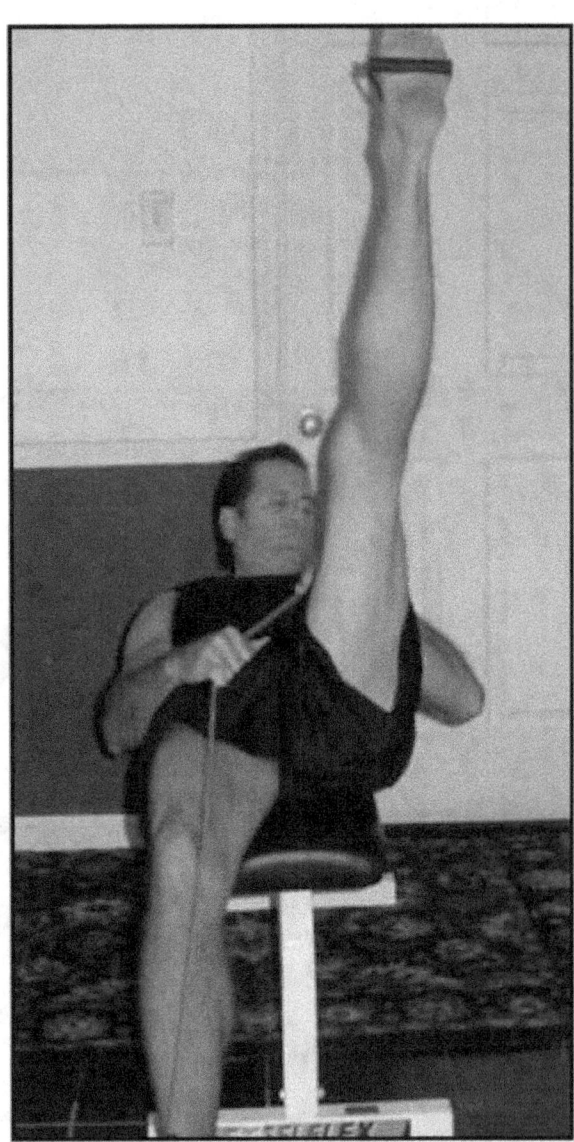 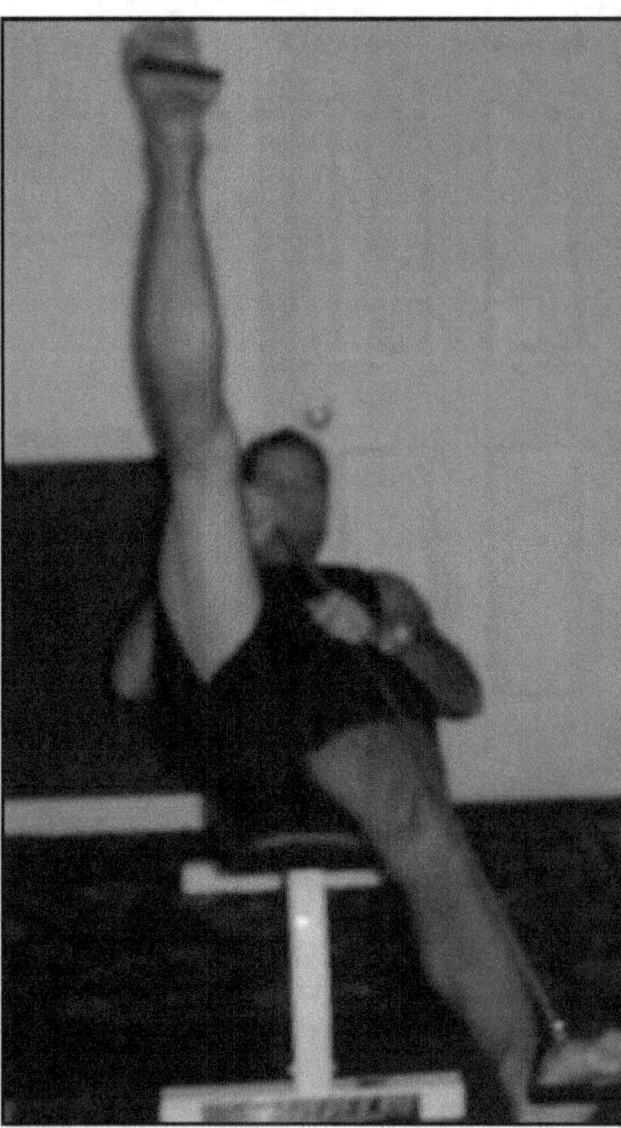

This is a variation of the leg lift
were we alternate legs, first
lifting one then the other. .

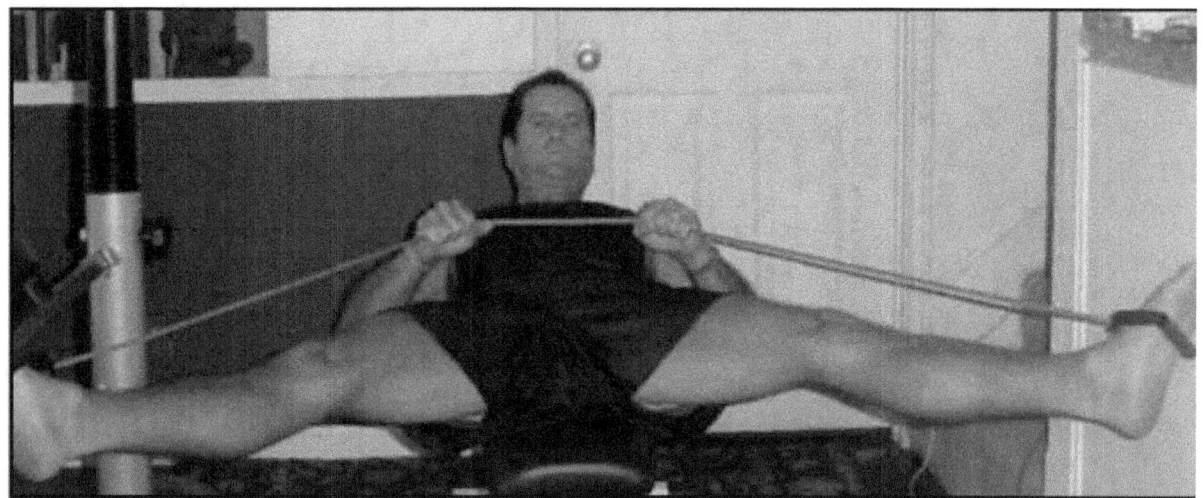

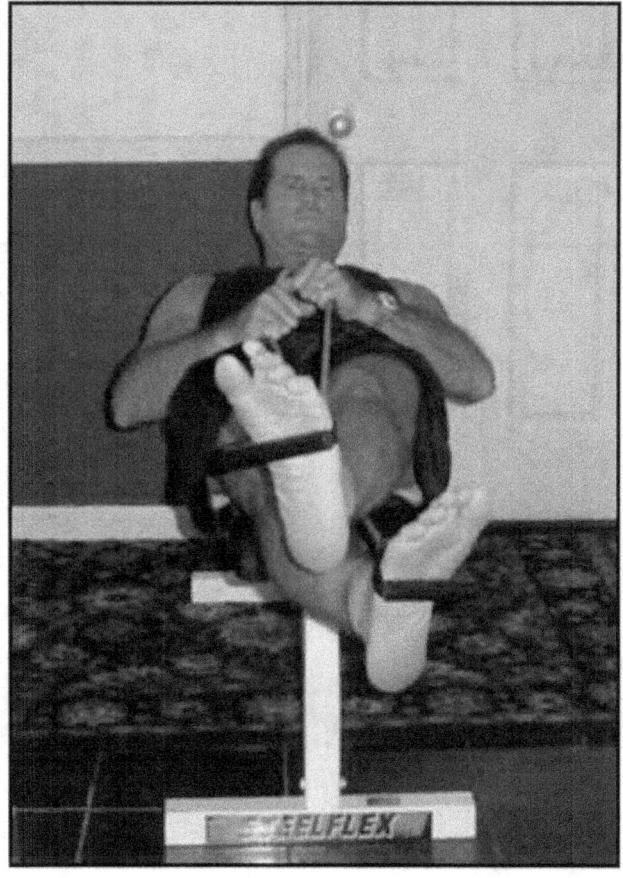

Here we start with the legs out fully extended to the side, then we being them together and over each other, alternating which leg goes on top with each movement. .

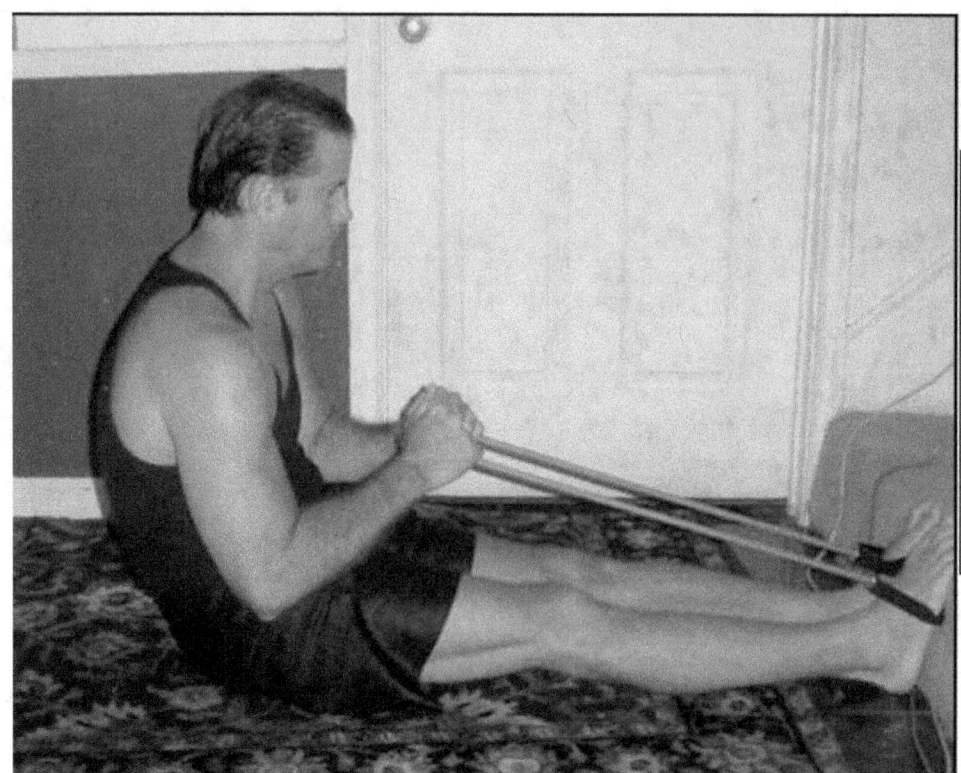

This is a sit up with the legs holding the tube and held against a wall for support, then we simply lean back and the up . .

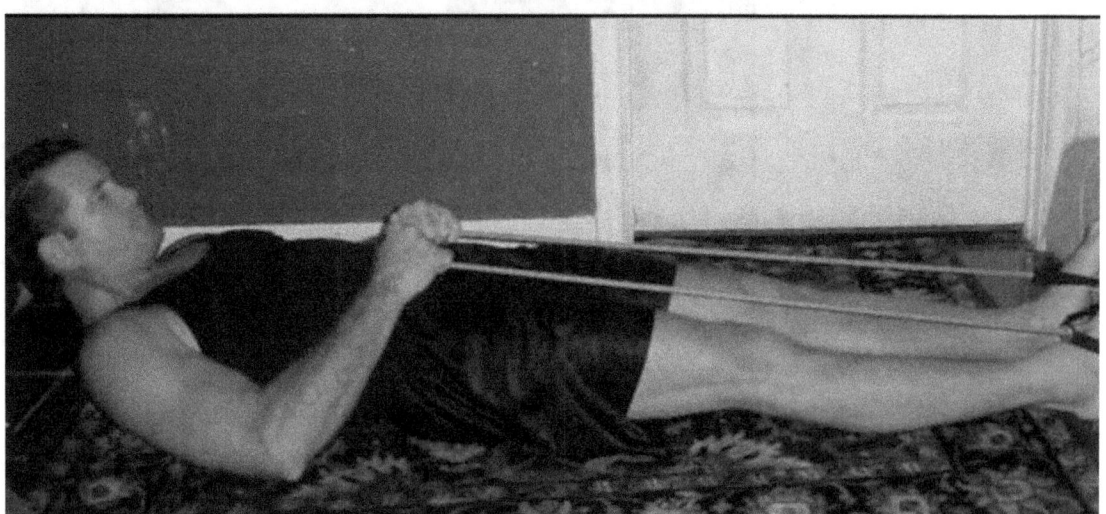

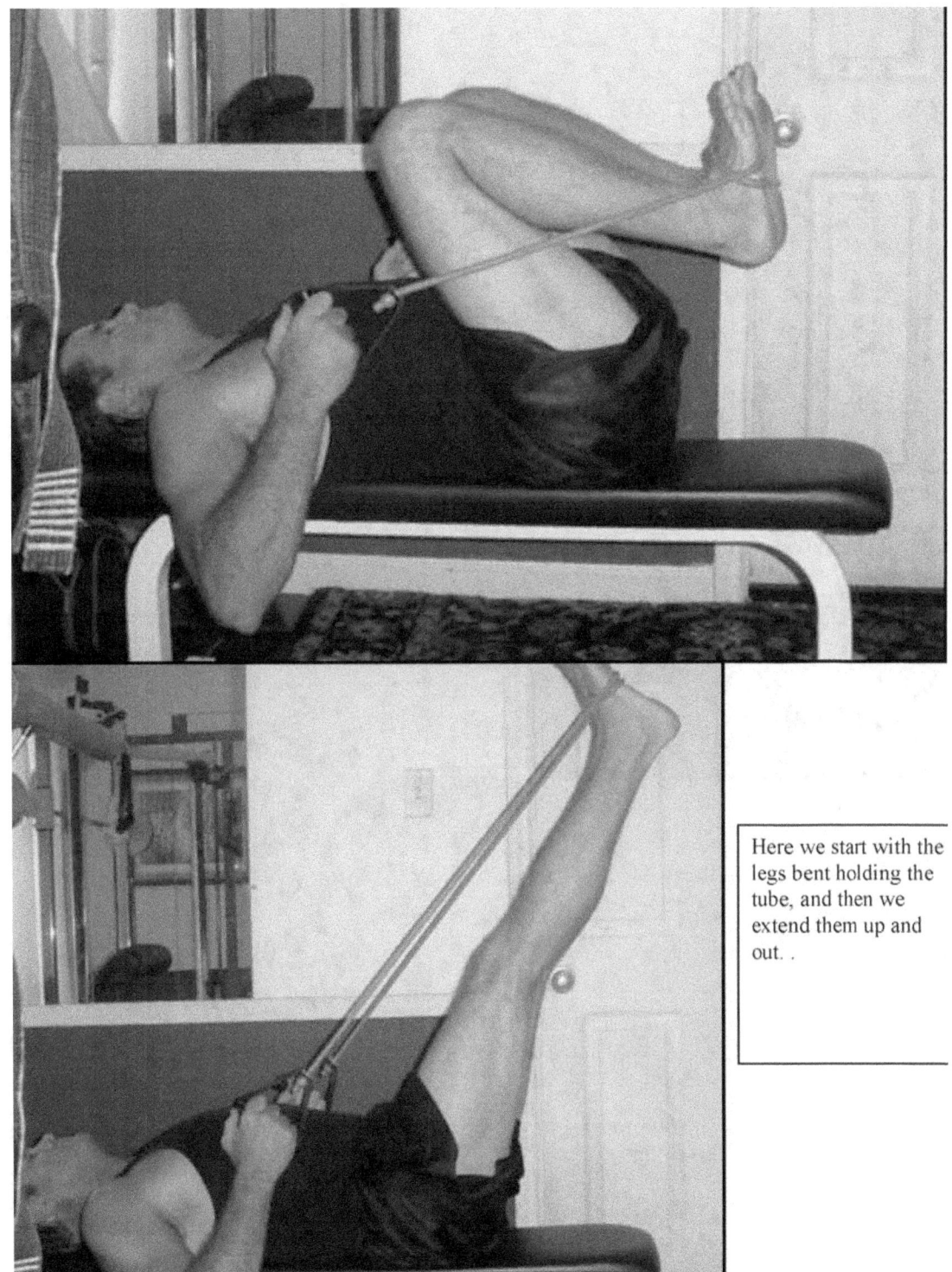

Here we start with the legs bent holding the tube, and then we extend them up and out. .

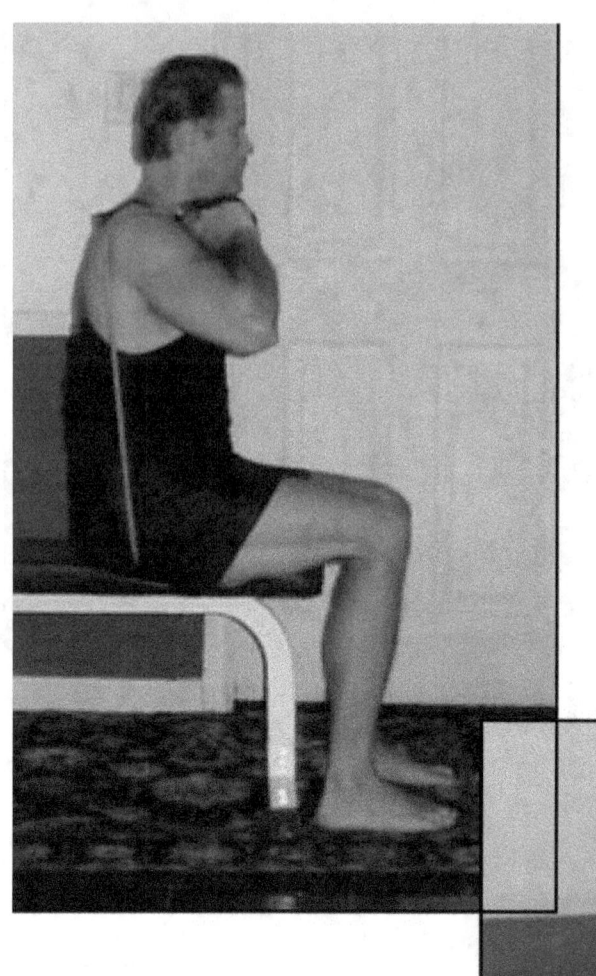

This is a sit down, we hold the tube up across our shoulders by sitting one it, then we simply lean down and forward to do the move.

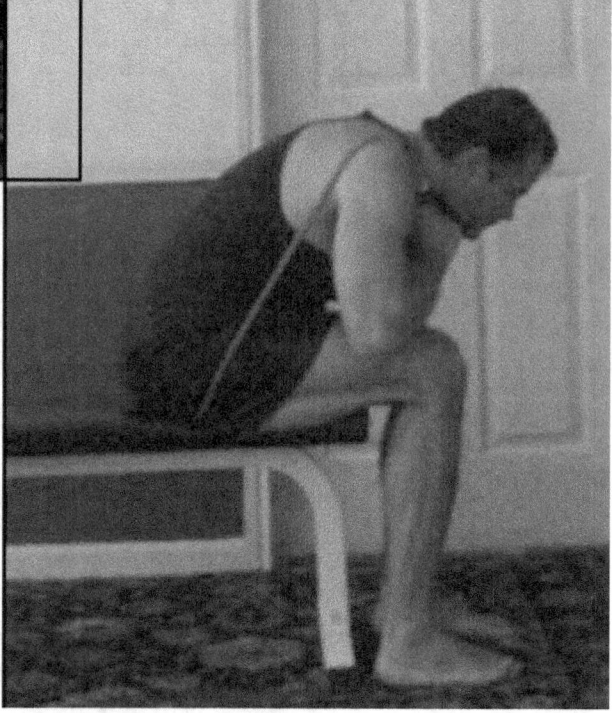

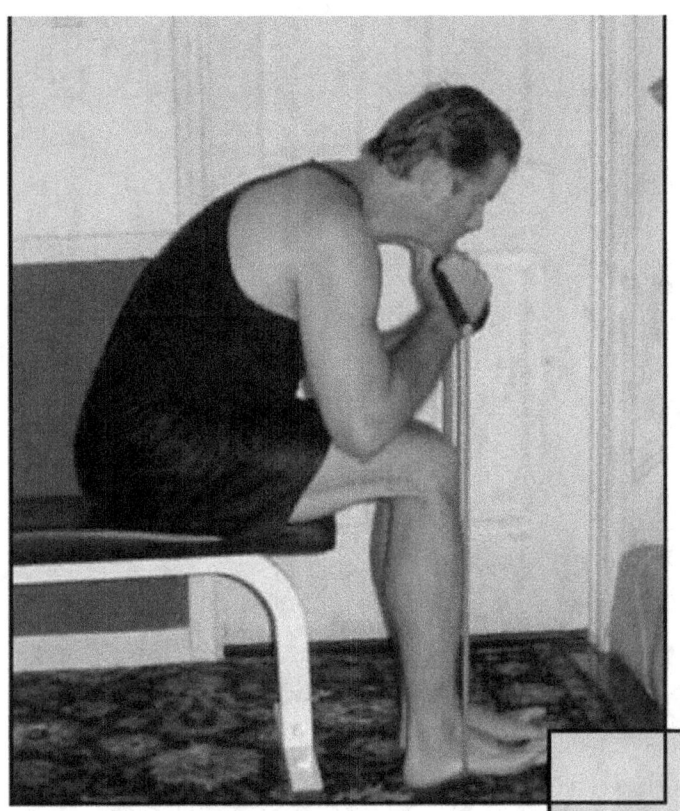

This is a sit back, we hold the tube to our chin, while leaning down, then the we pull our body up straight. .

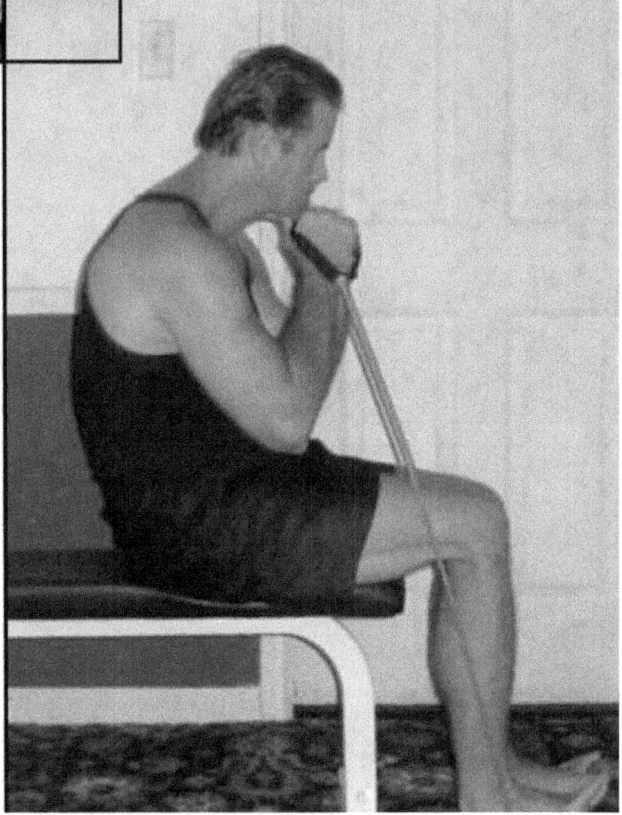

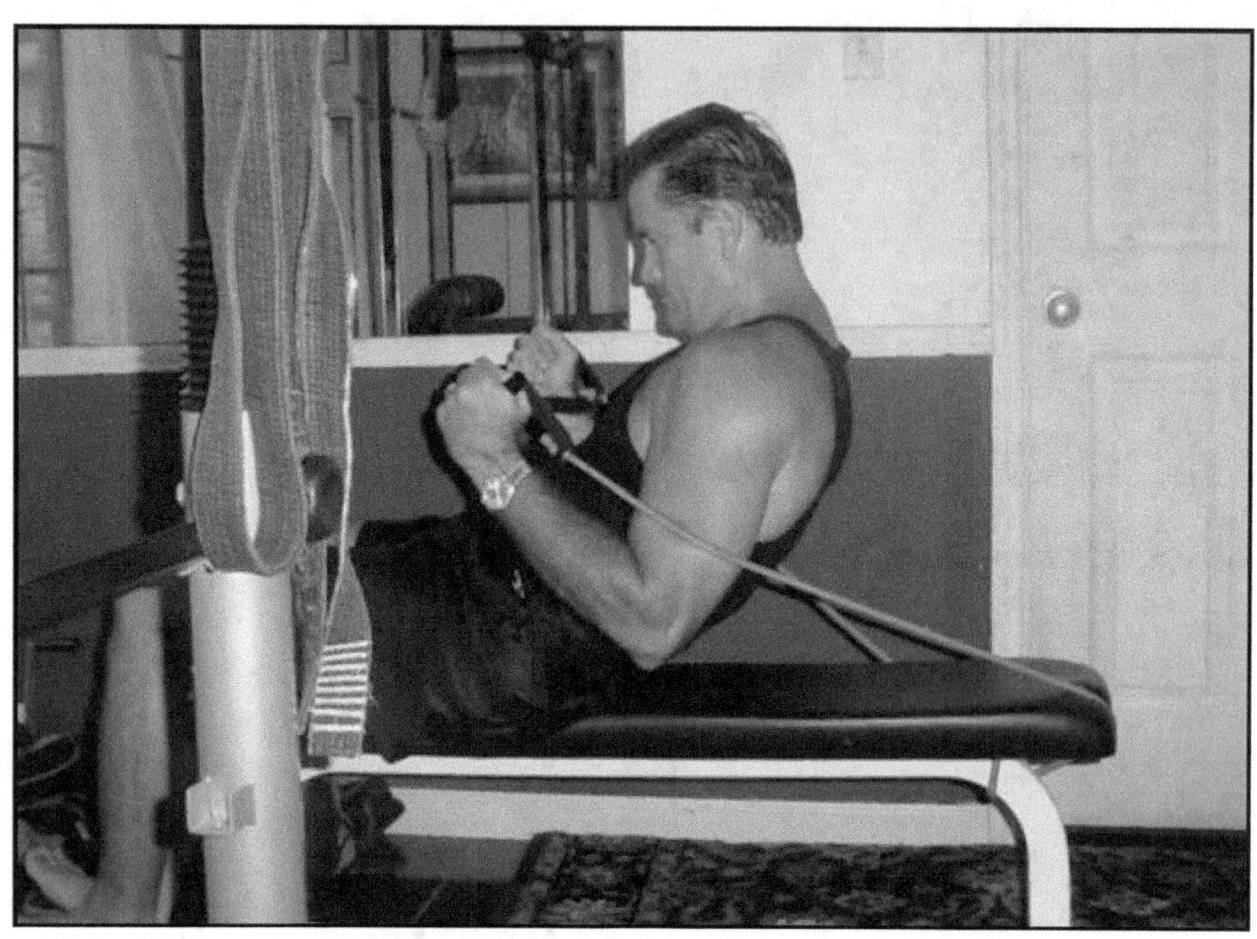

This is a sit up done
with the tube wrapped
around the back of the
bench.

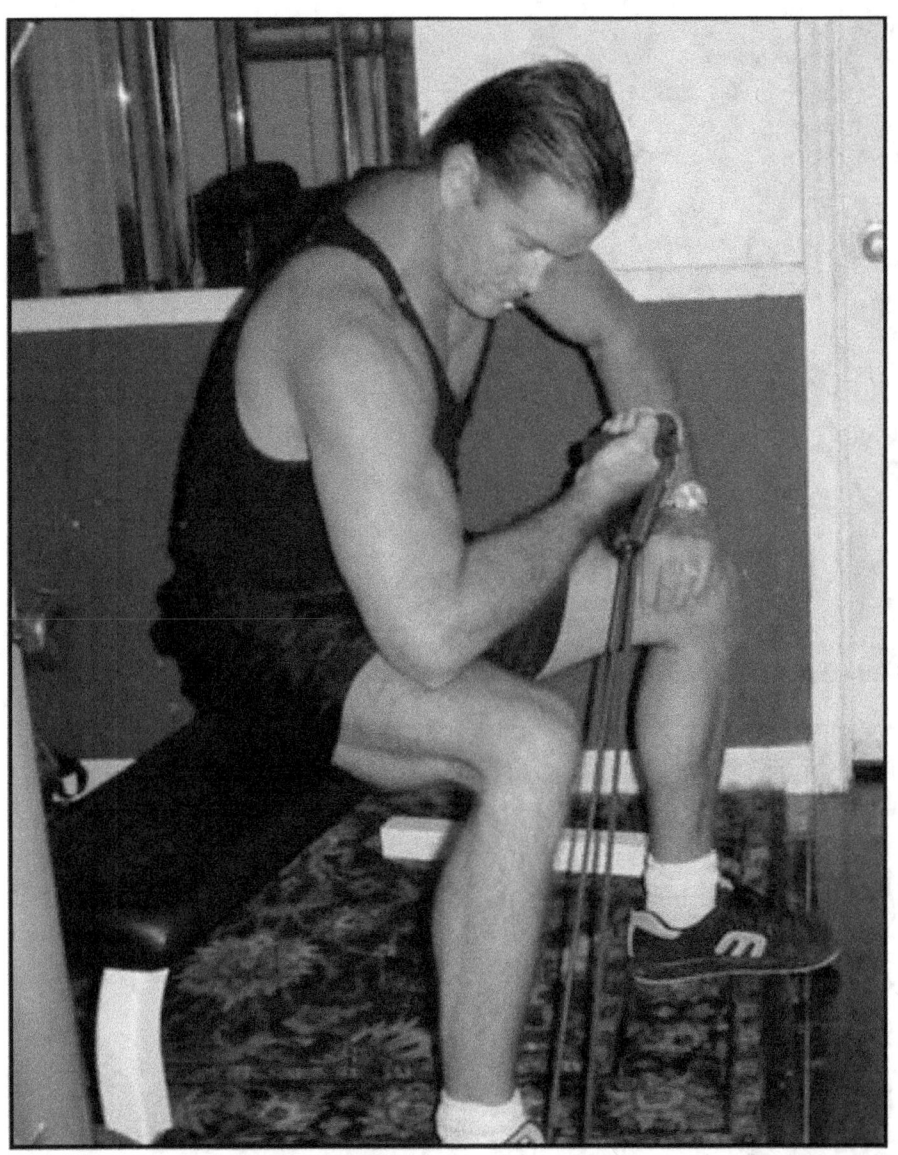

Here we work the
biceps by sitting down
and having the arm sit
on top of our knee then
pulling the arm up.

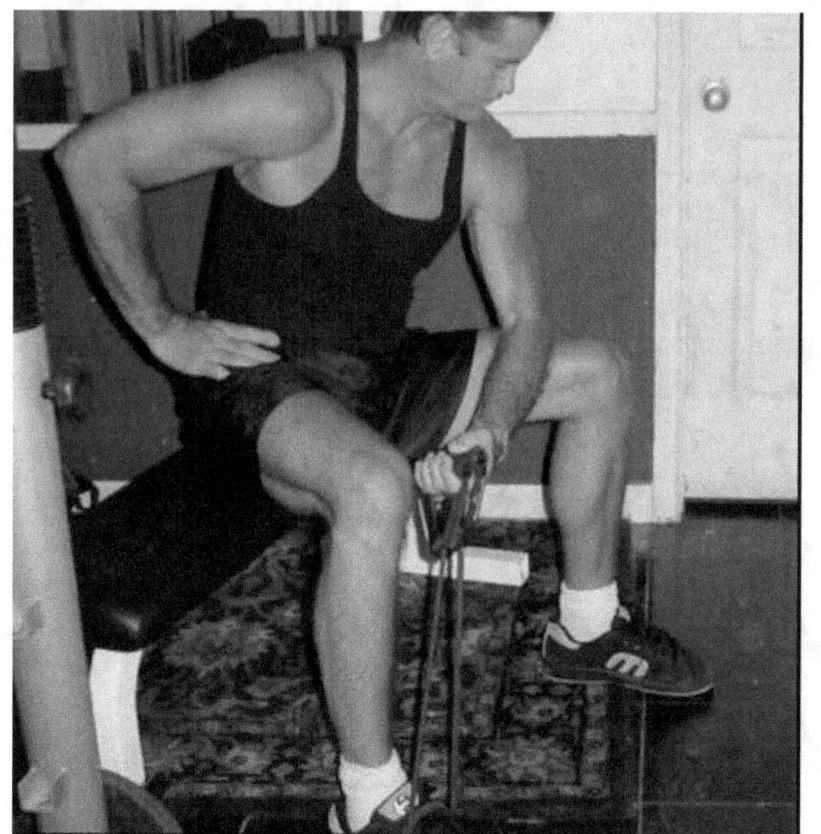

Here we work the biceps sitting down with the arm on top of our knee, then lifting up to the chest.

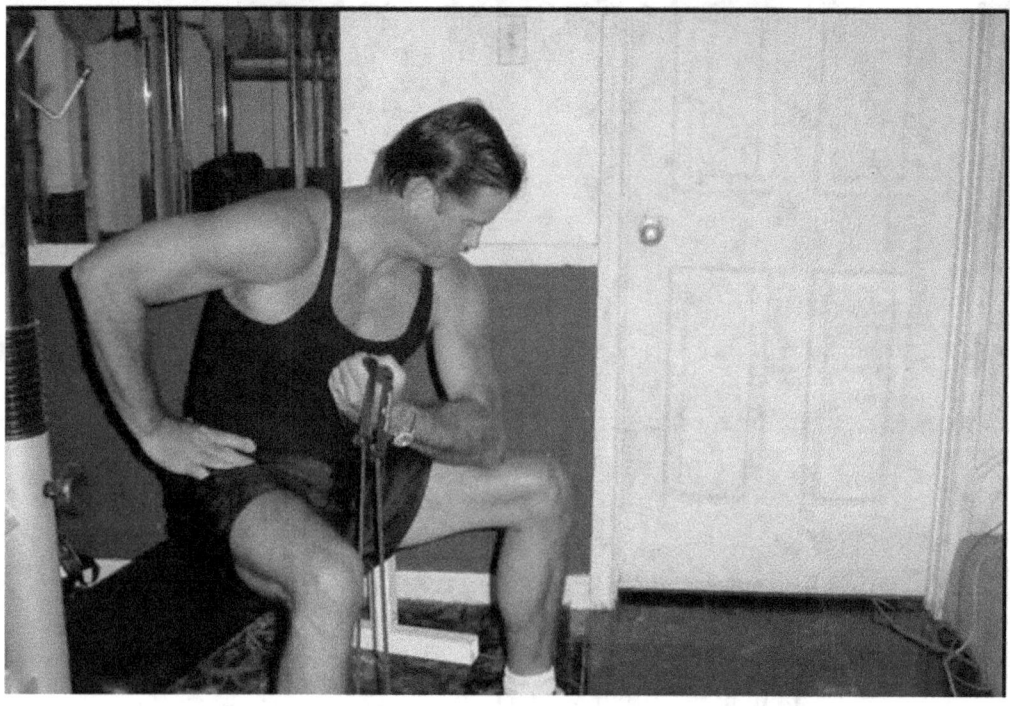

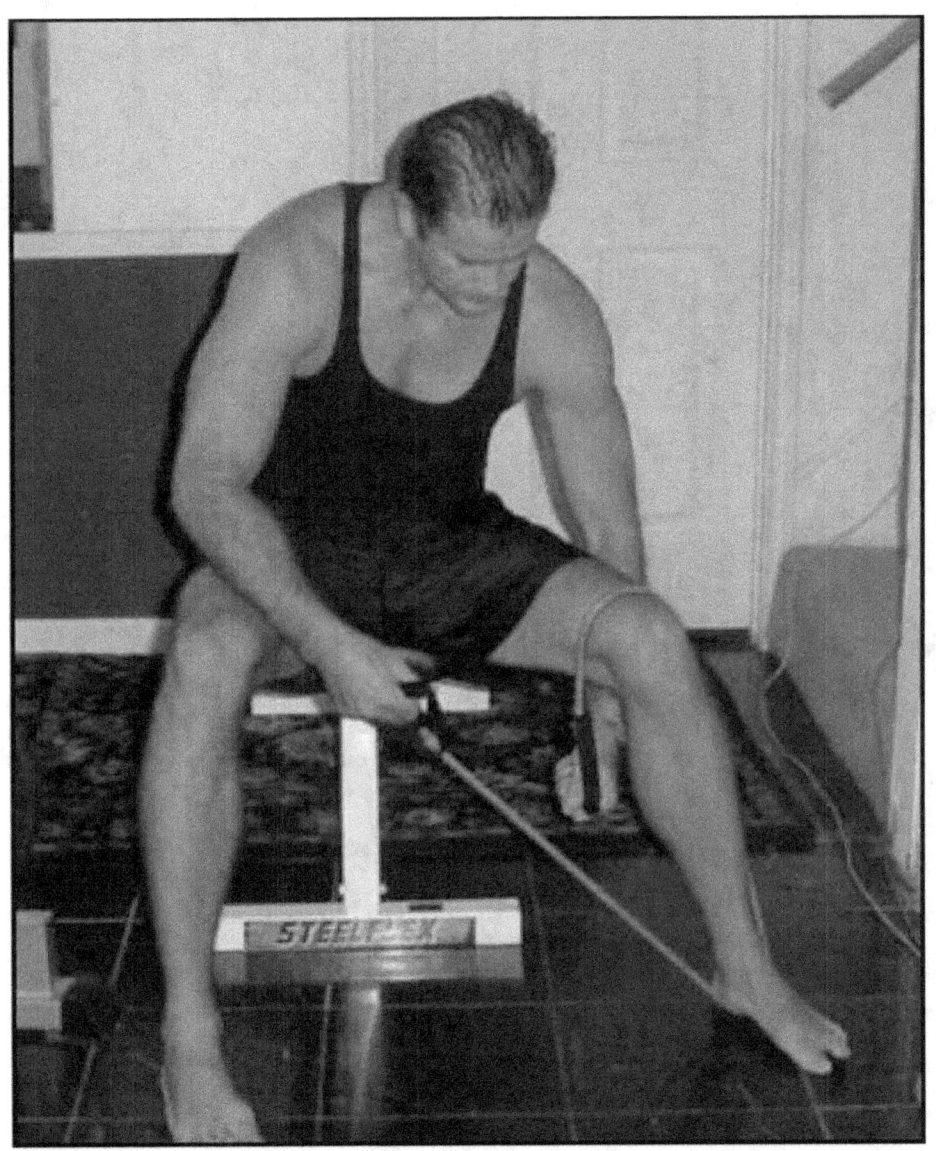

Here I show how to
wrap the tube around
my leg for exercising.

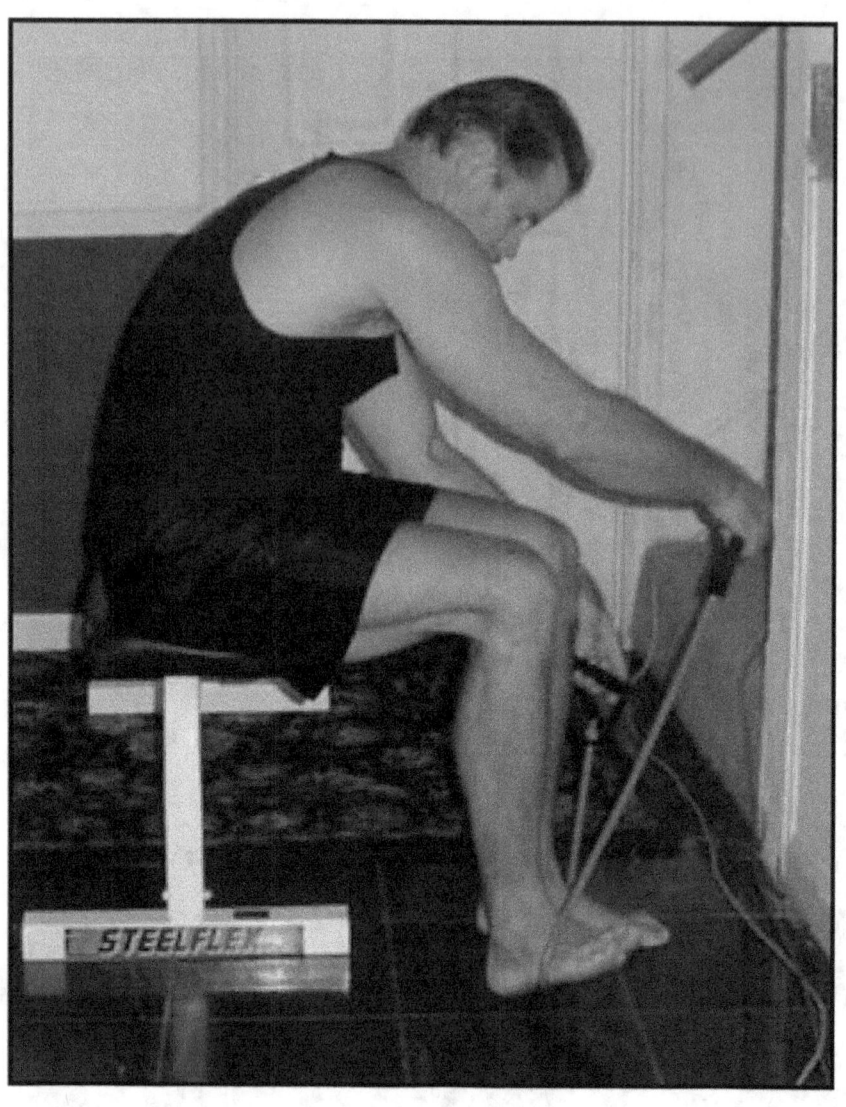

Here I show how to wrap the feet
around the tube for exercising.

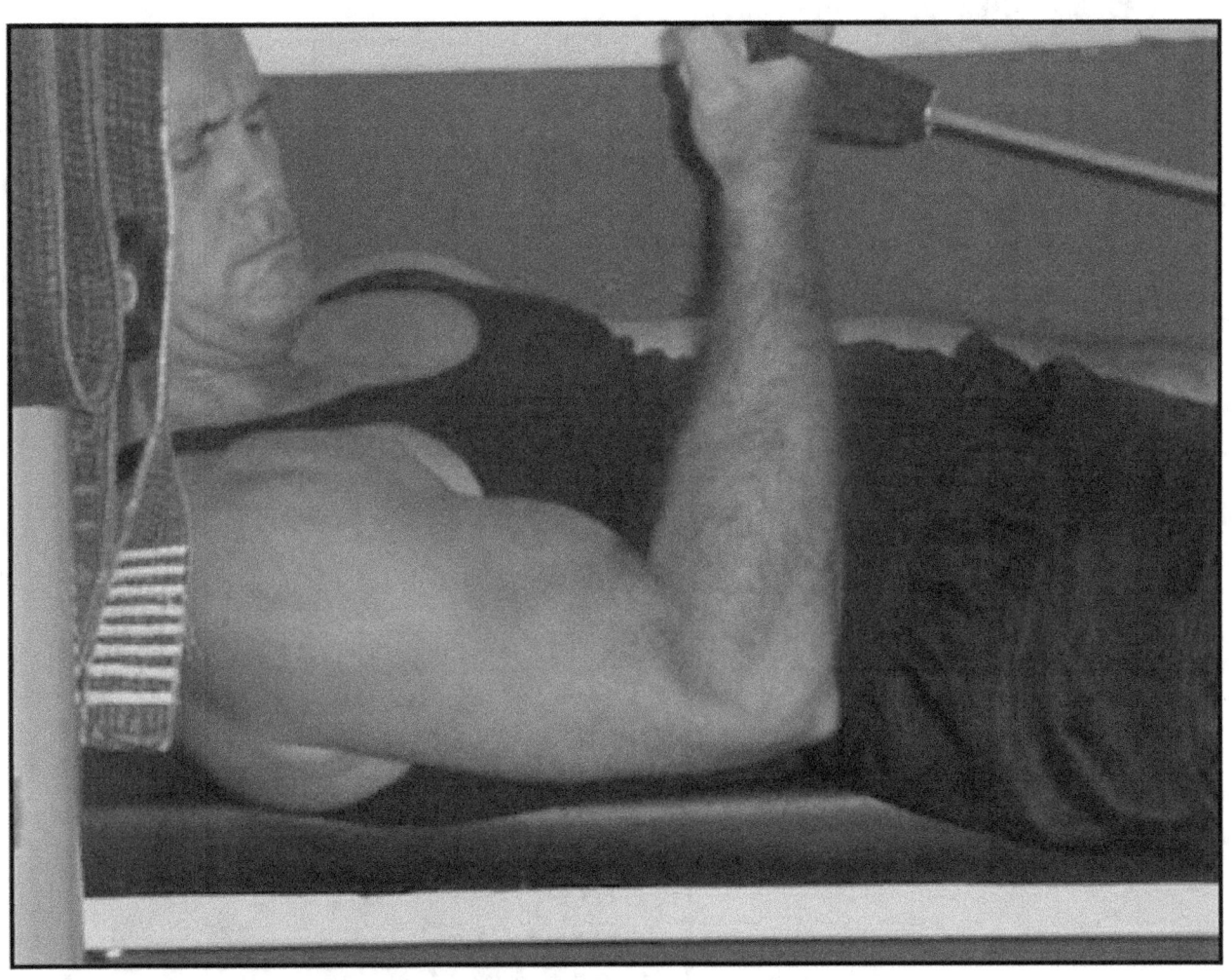

To get the most effect
from the exercise
really concentrate the
mind of the muscle
you are working. .

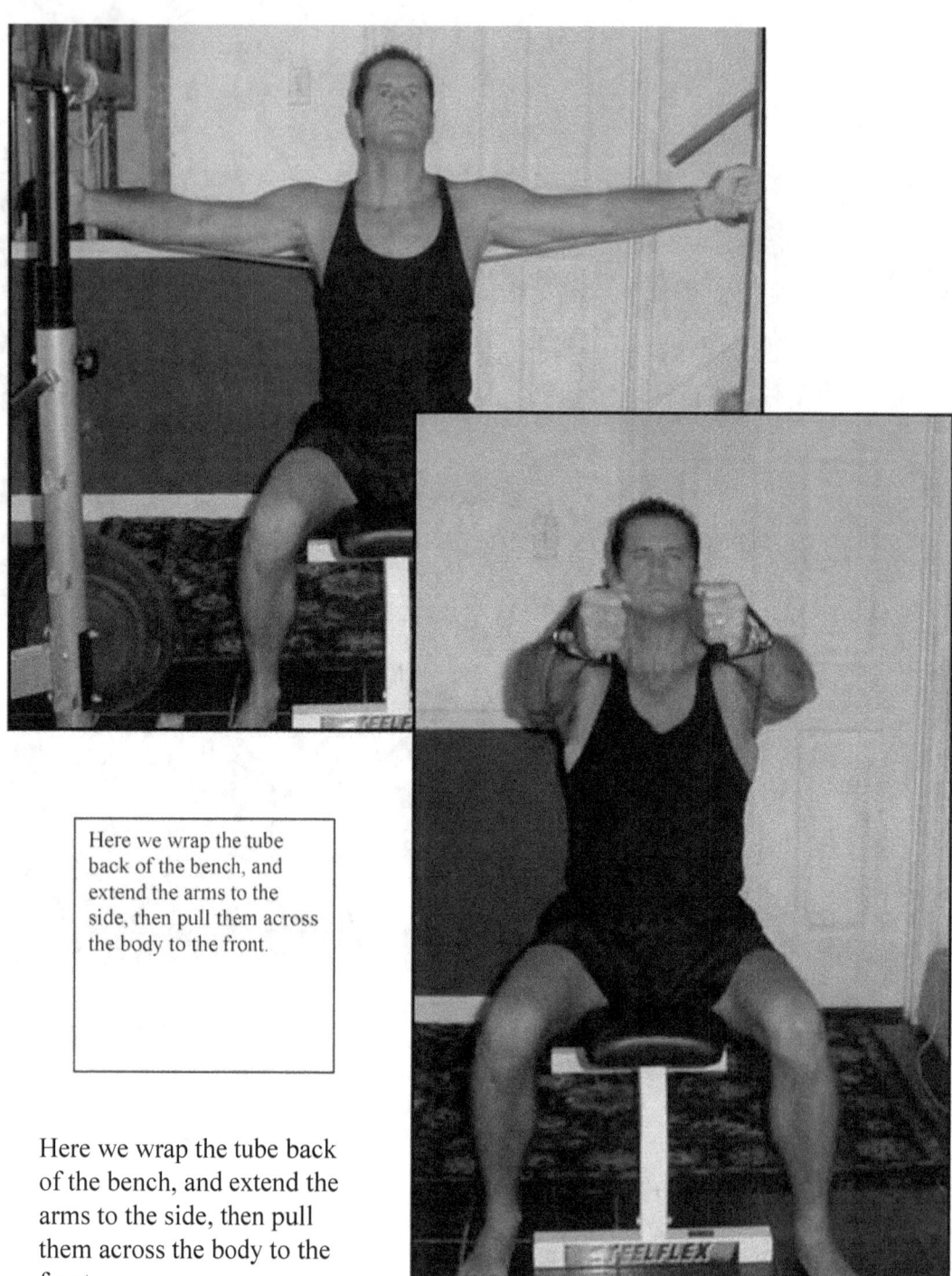

Here we wrap the tube
back of the bench, and
extend the arms to the
side, then pull them across
the body to the front.

Here we wrap the tube back
of the bench, and extend the
arms to the side, then pull
them across the body to the
front.

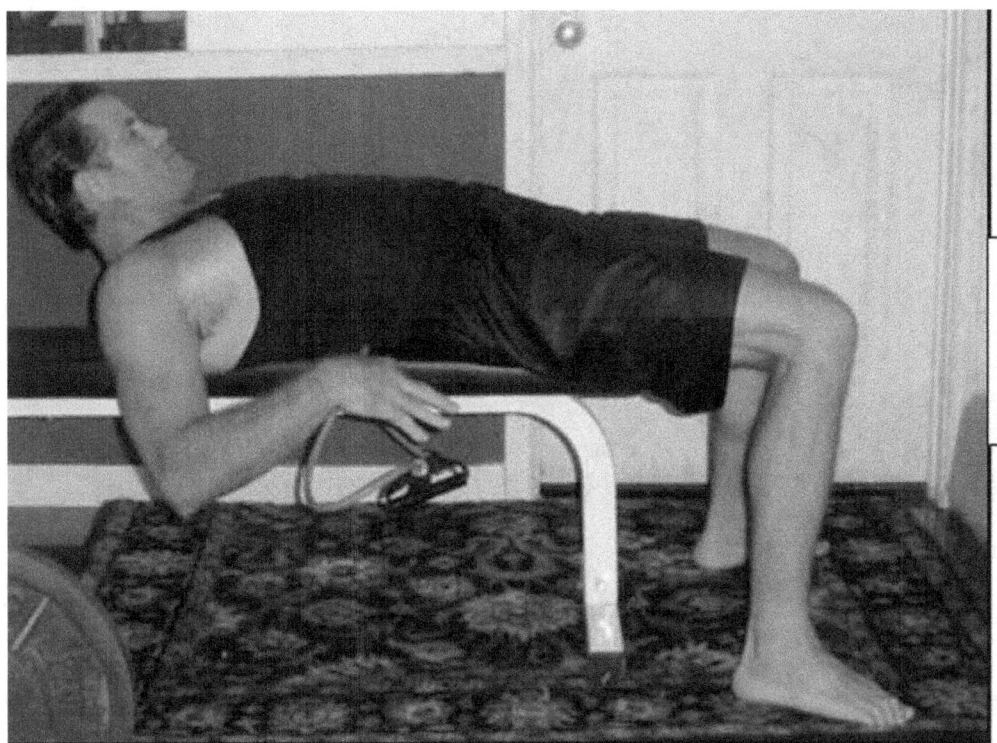

Here we wrap the tube under the bench and do a regular bench press.

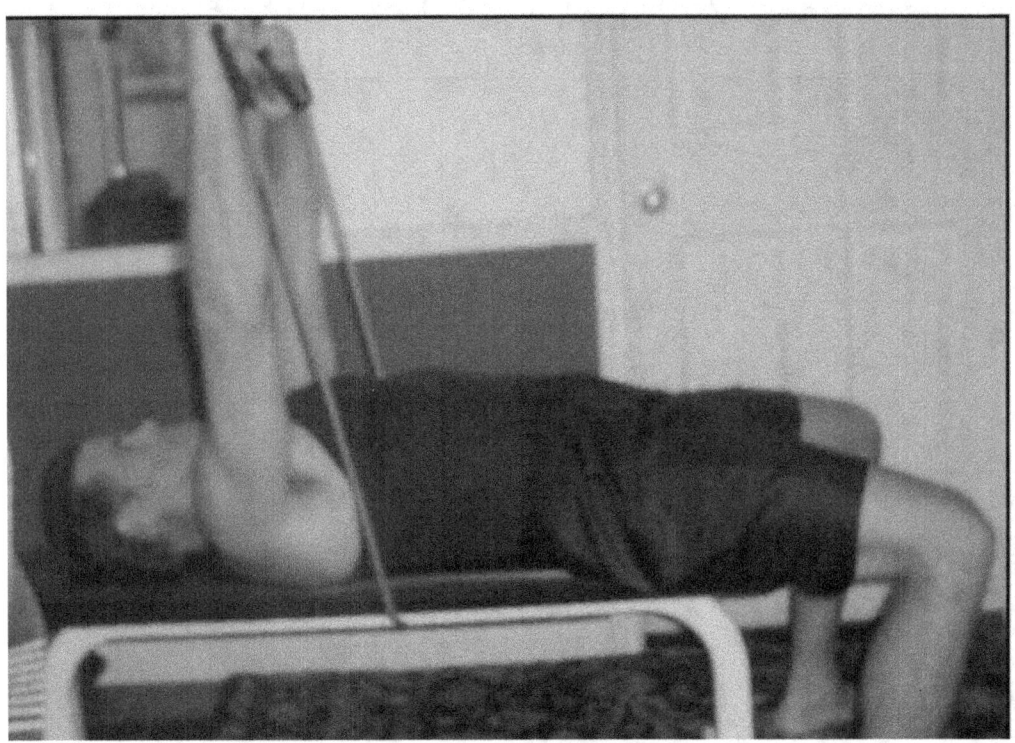

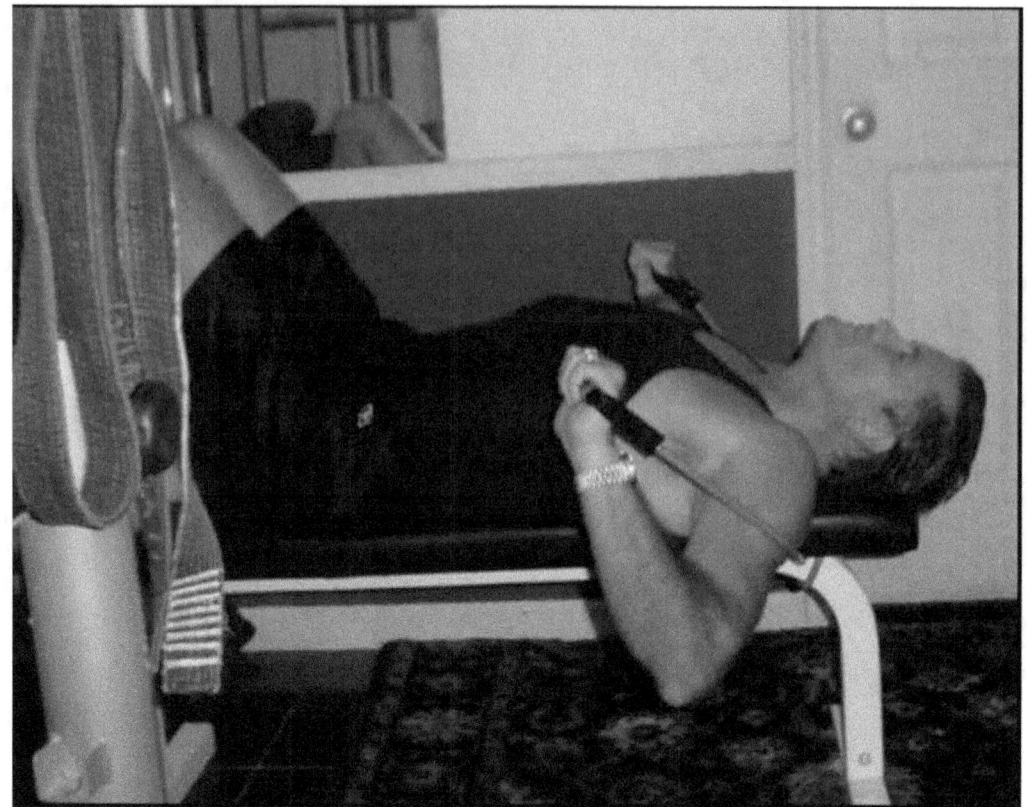

Here we wrap
the tube under
the do a bench
press forward
and out to
work the lower
chest. .

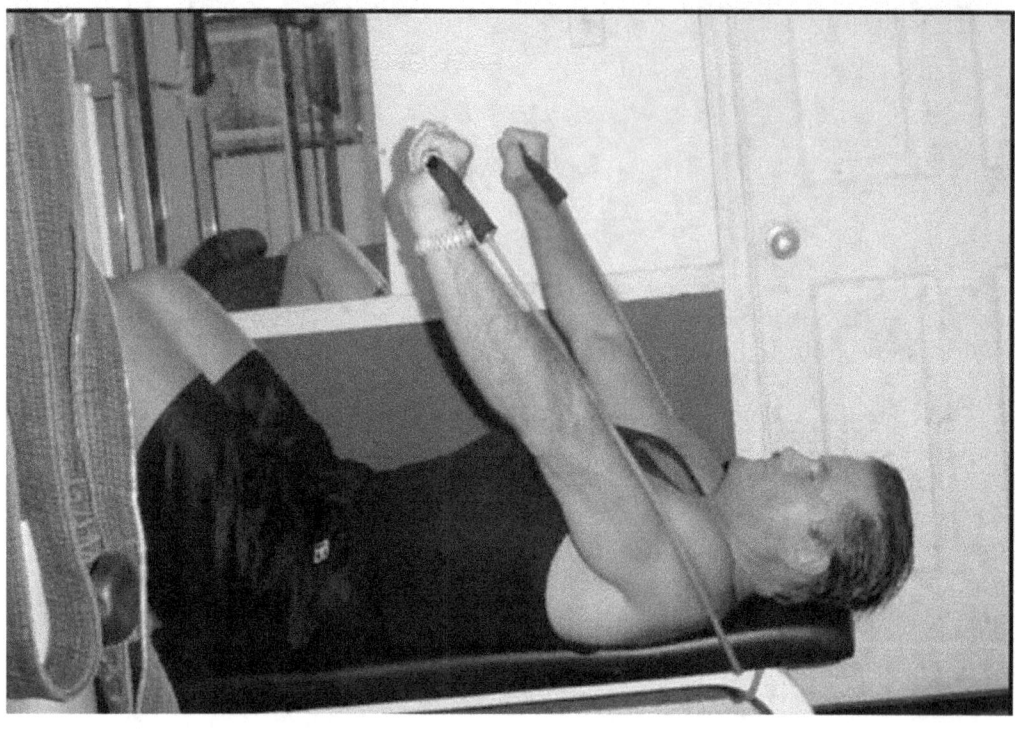

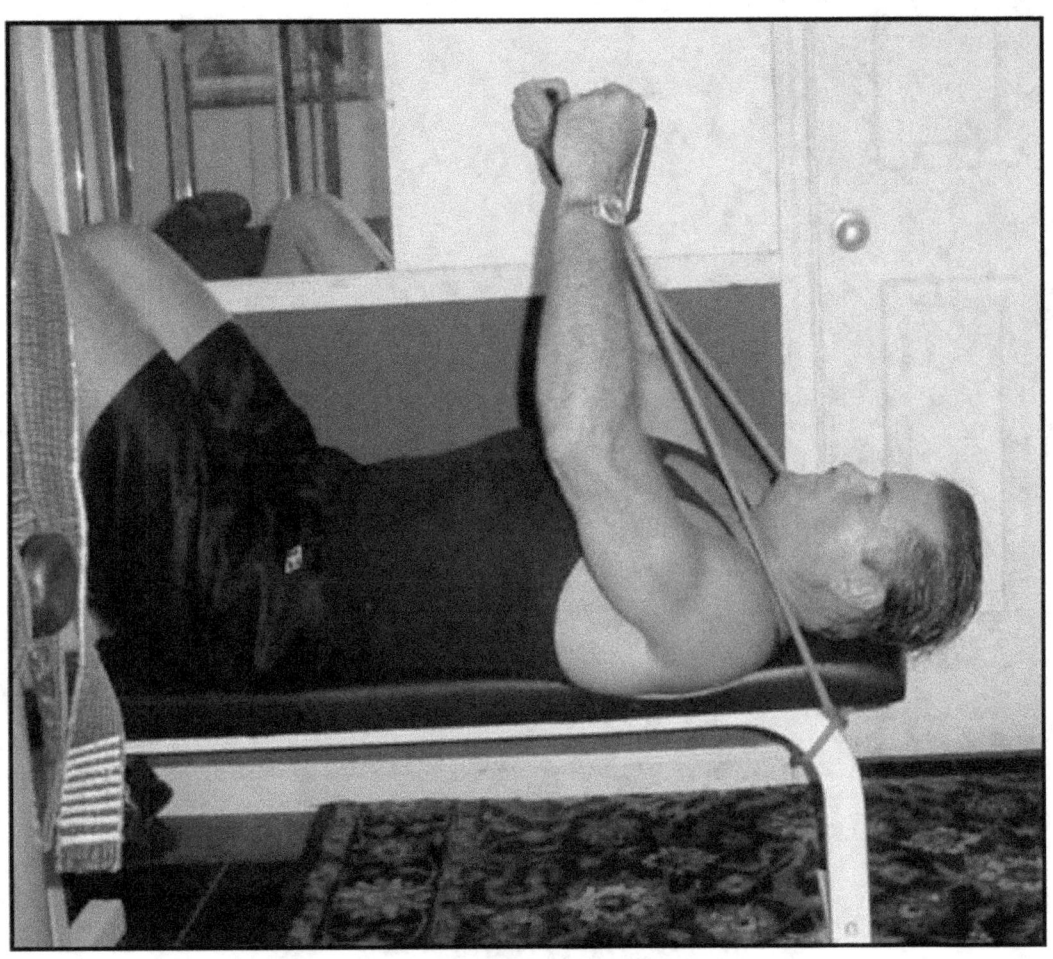

Here we wrap the tube
under the bench and do
a regular bench press.,
but this time we cross
the tube in front of our
body.

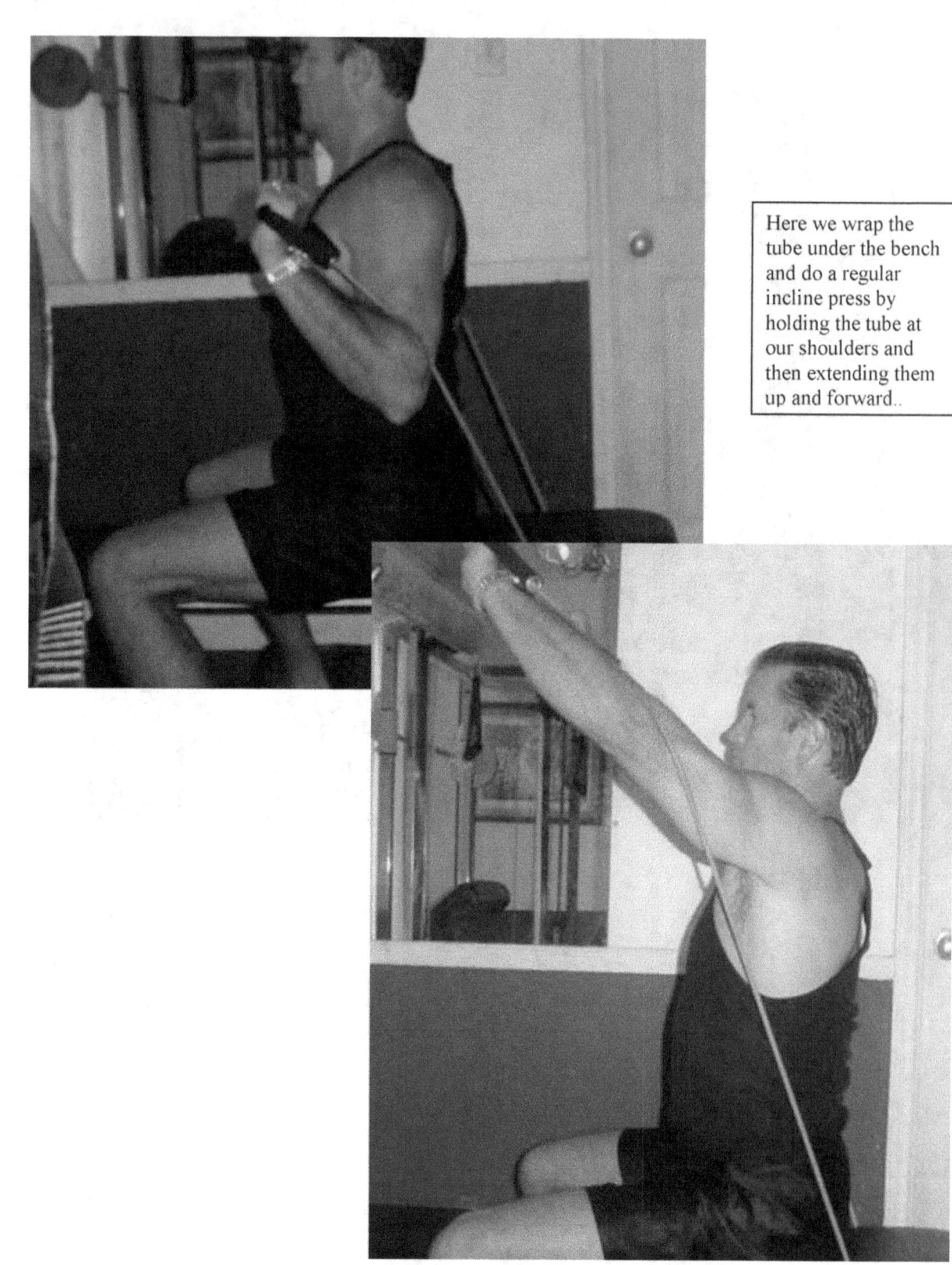

Here we wrap the tube under the bench and do a regular incline press by holding the tube at our shoulders and then extending them up and forward..

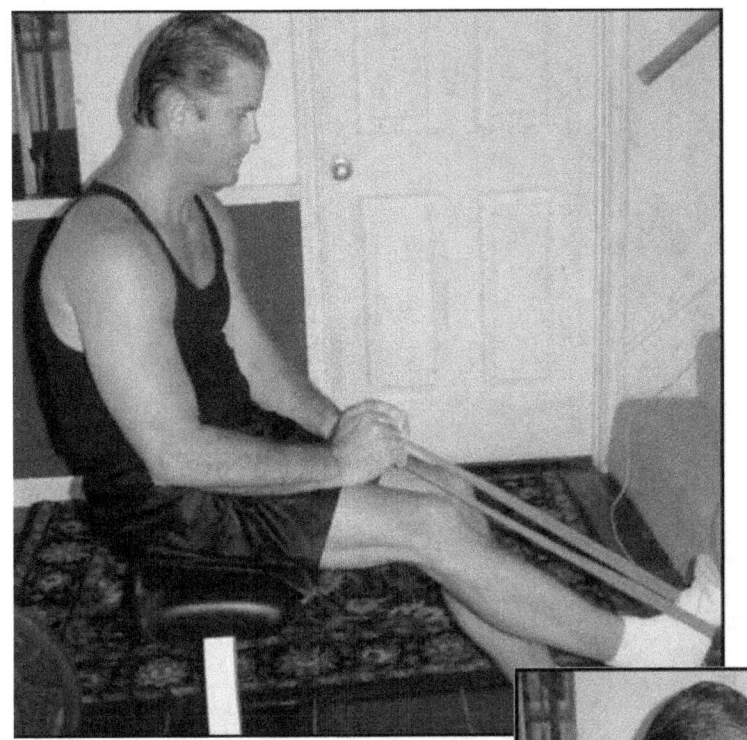

Here we hold the tube on our foot work the ankle and calf, by extending the ankle.

This is the same exercise done without a sock for a more secure hold.

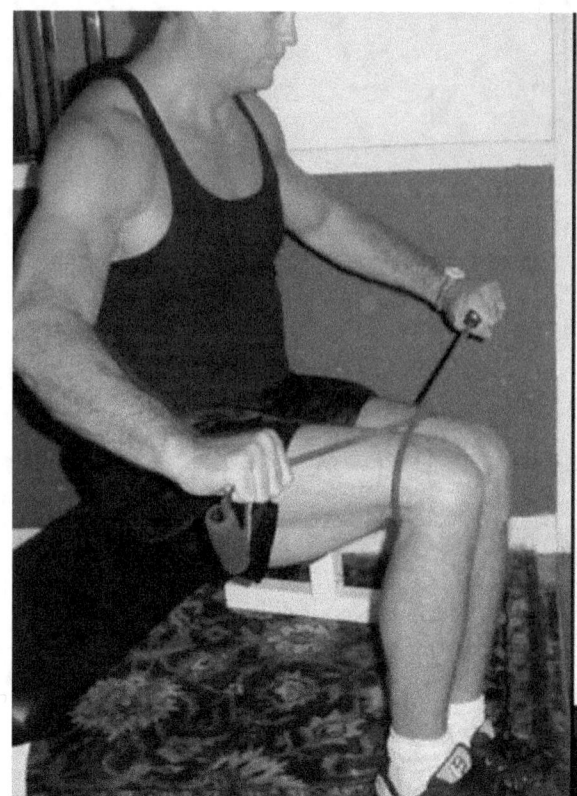

Here we work the inner thigh by wrapping the tube around knees the pulling the legs apart at the knees.

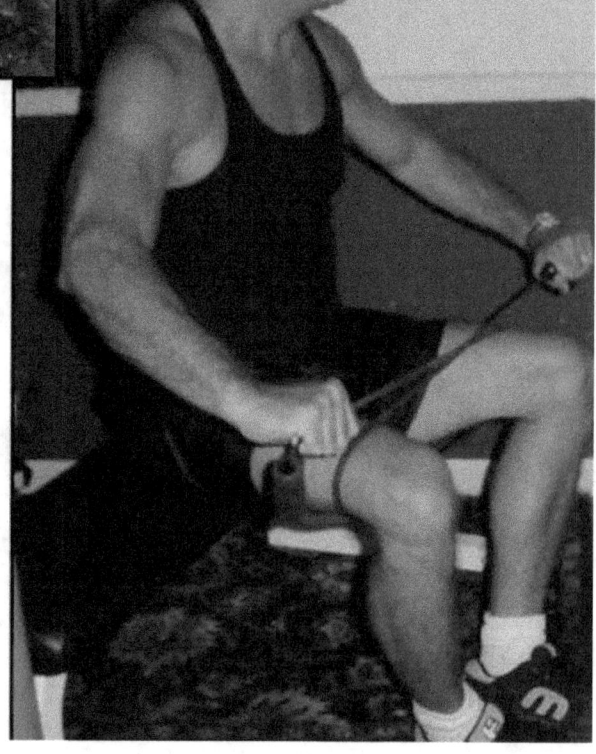

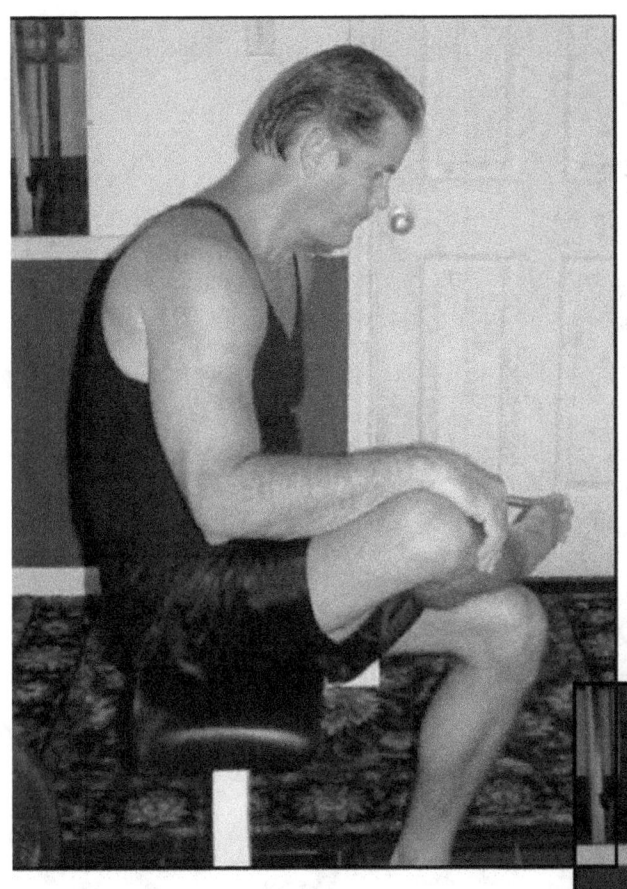

Here we work
the ankle by
wrapping the
tube around
the foot and
then flexing it.

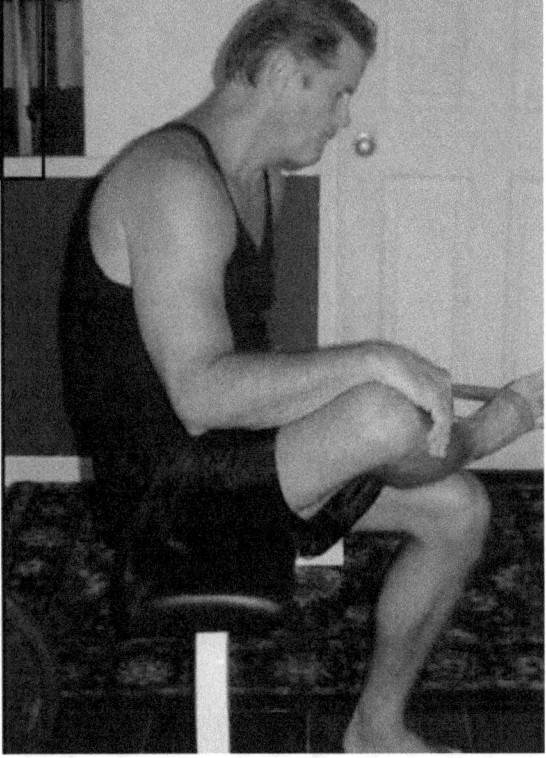

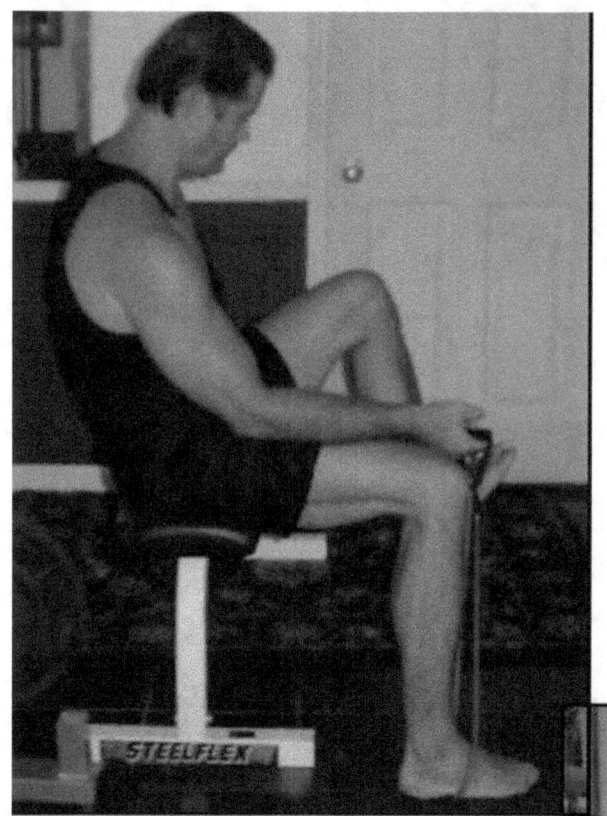

Here we hold the tube wrapped around out foot and held by the other foot with the leg bent, then we extend the foot forward.

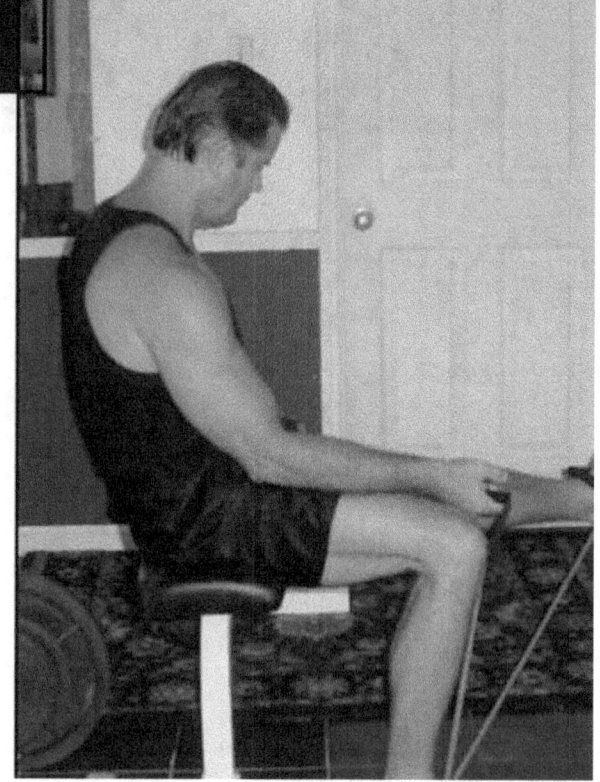

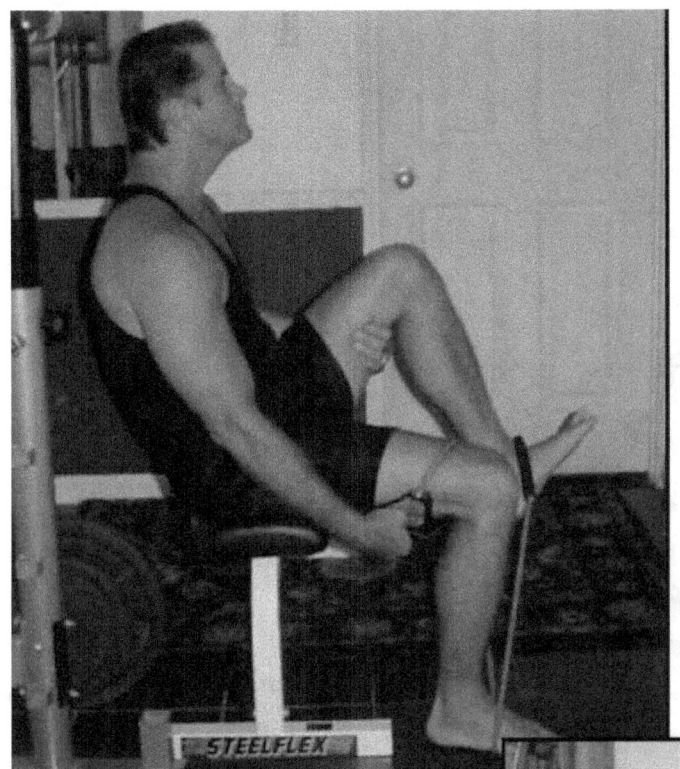

Here we hold the tube wrapped around out foot and held by the other foot with the leg bent, then we extend the foot forward. We hold the extending leg for support.

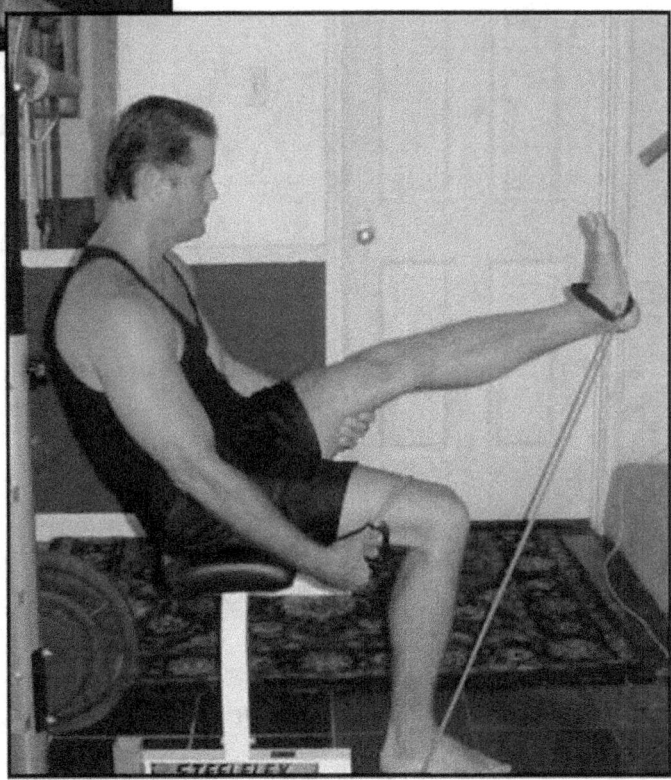

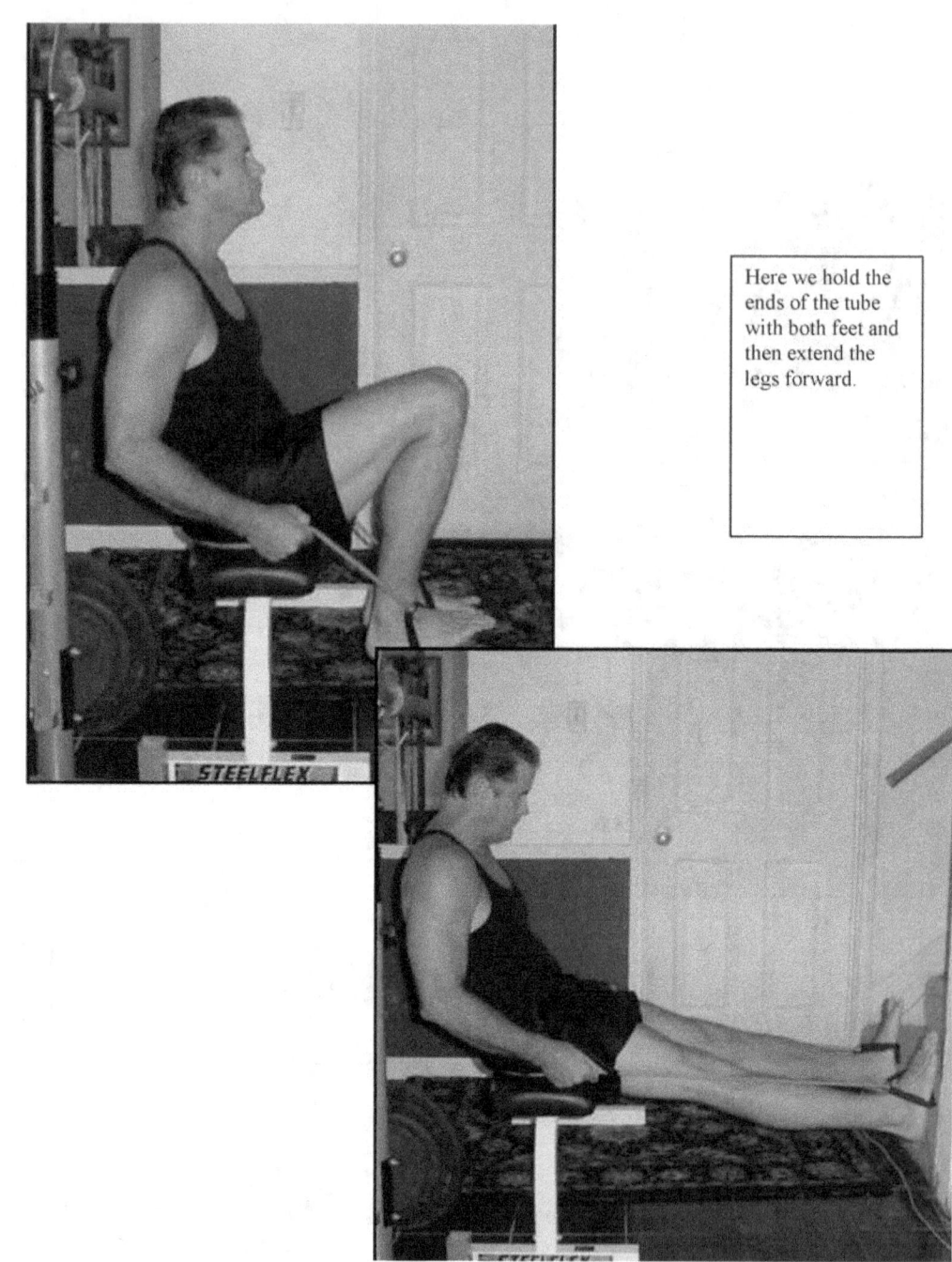

Here we hold the ends of the tube with both feet and then extend the legs forward.

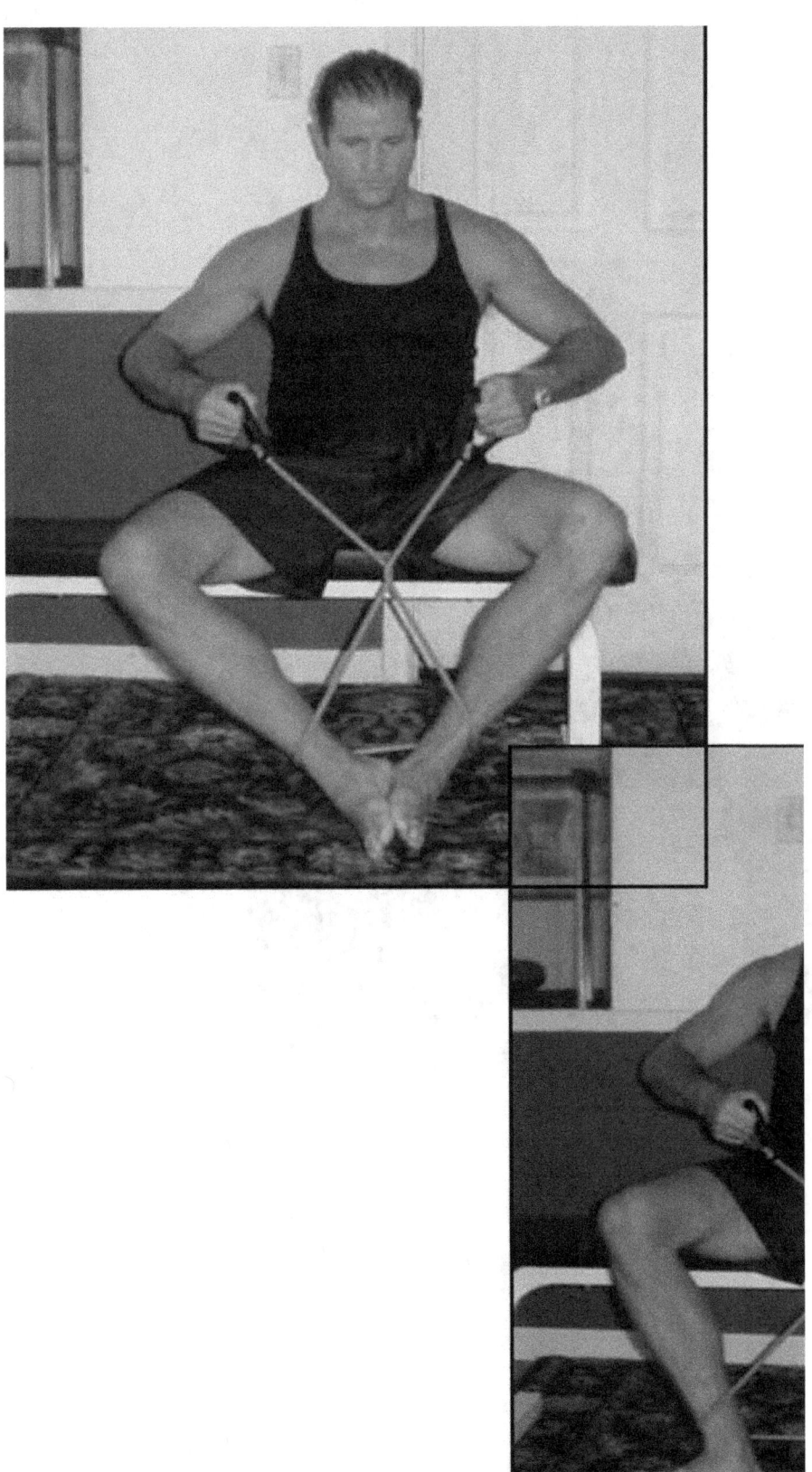

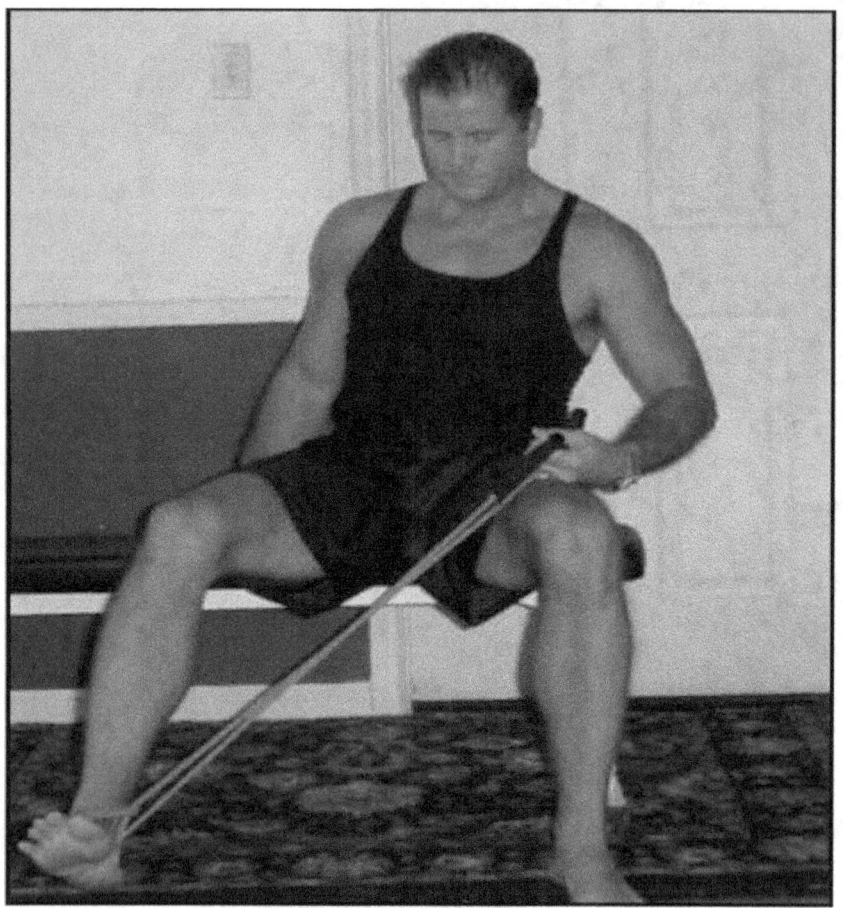

Here wrap the tube over the foot and pull the leg away from the bench.

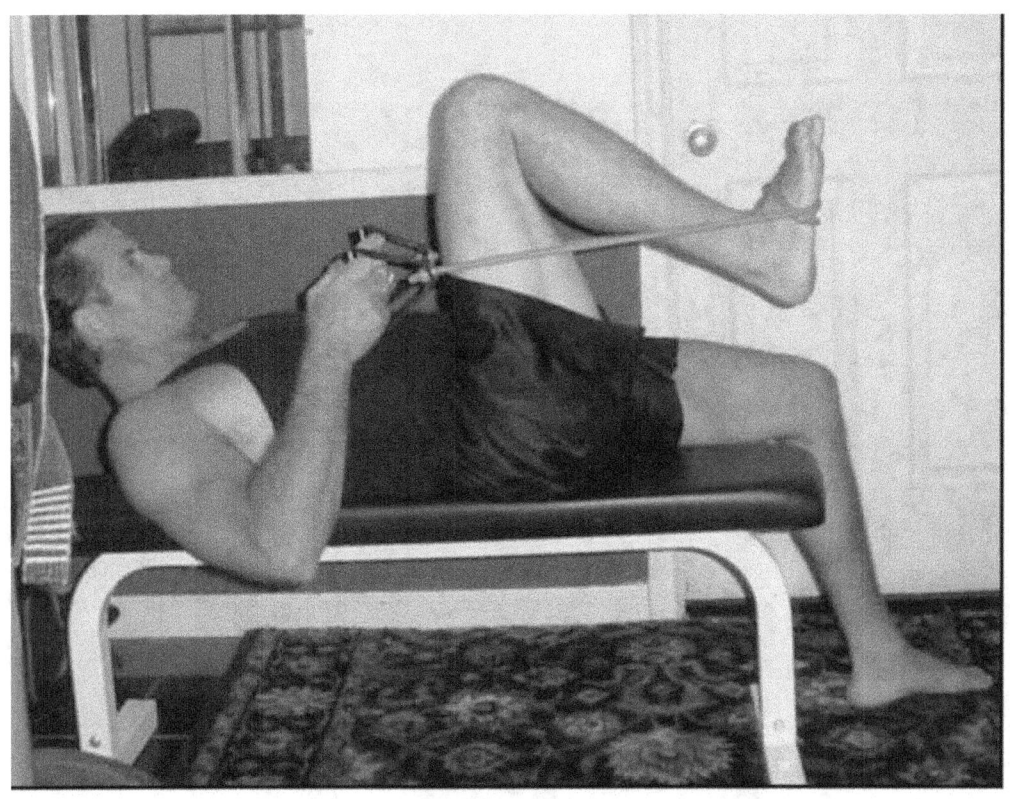

Here wrap the tube around the foot,
bending the leg and then extending it
directly out.

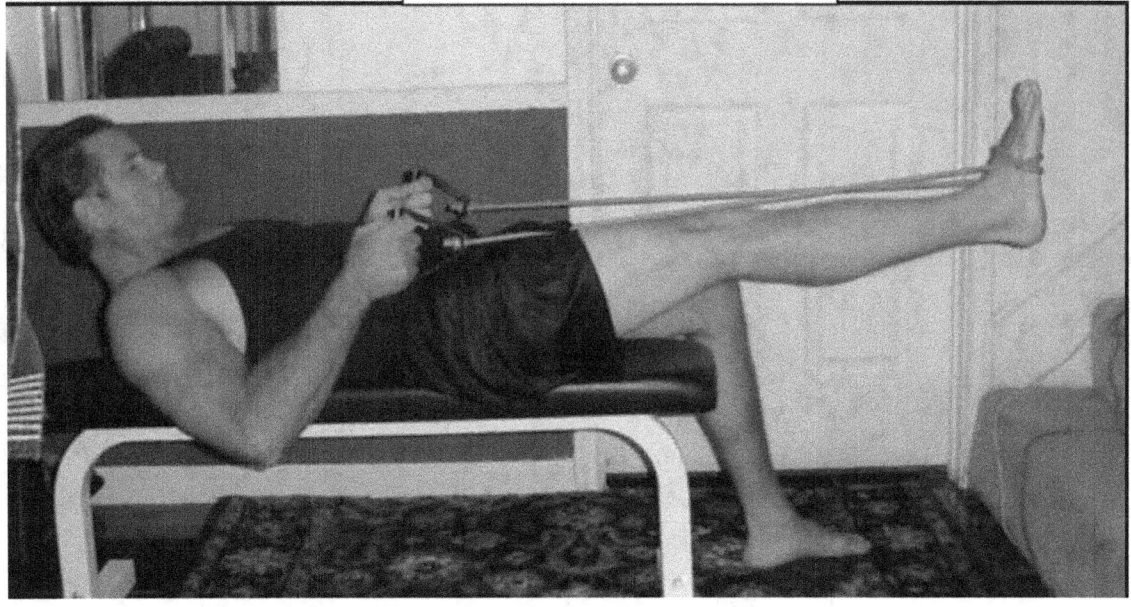

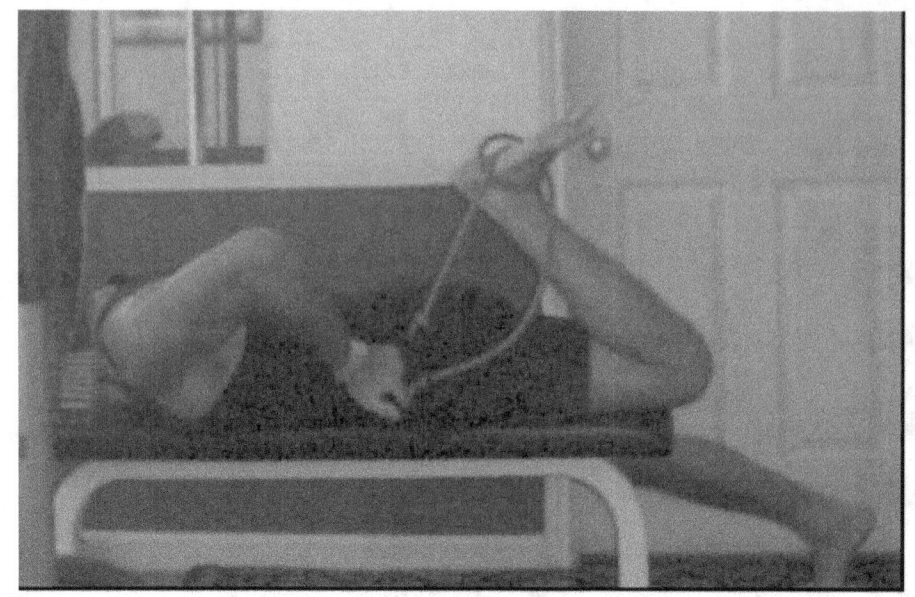

Here we wrap the tube around our foot, while lying face down on the bench, then extend the leg out and back.

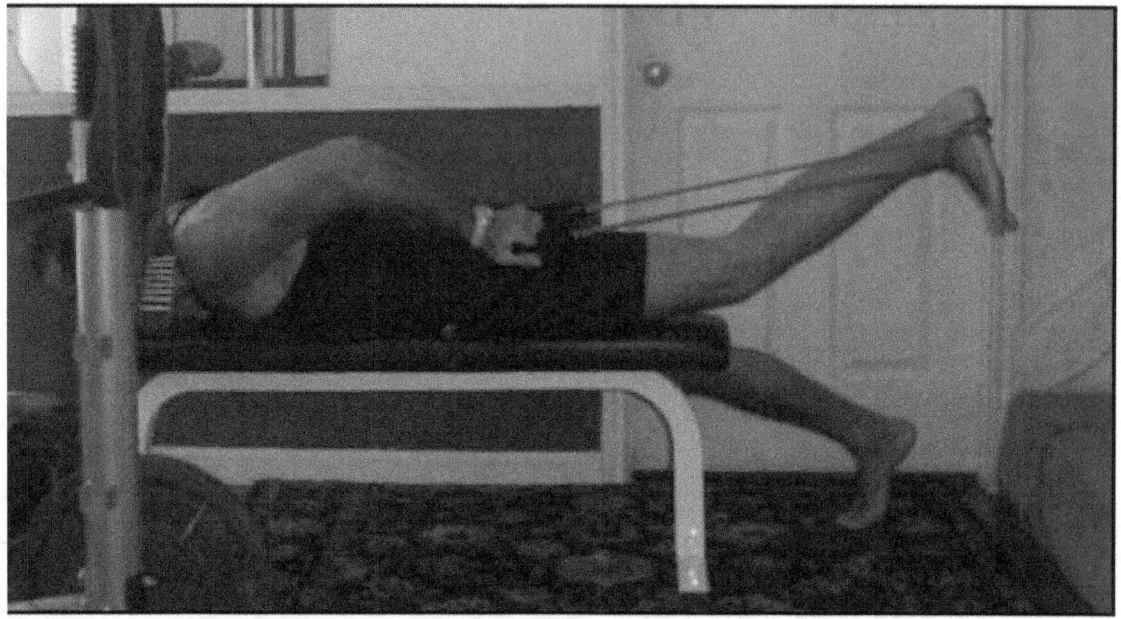

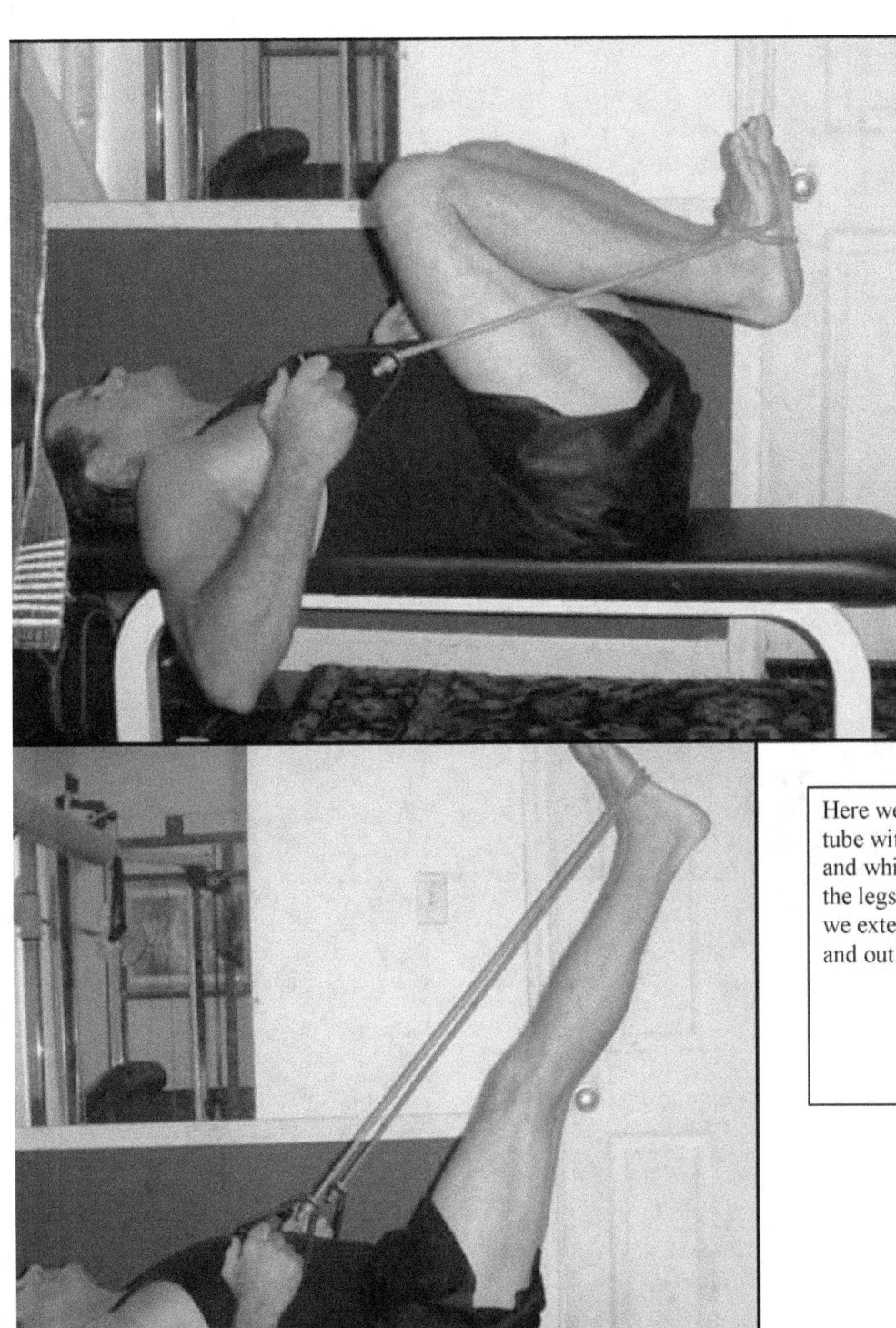

Here we hold th
tube with our fe
and while havin
the legs bent, th
we extend them
and out.

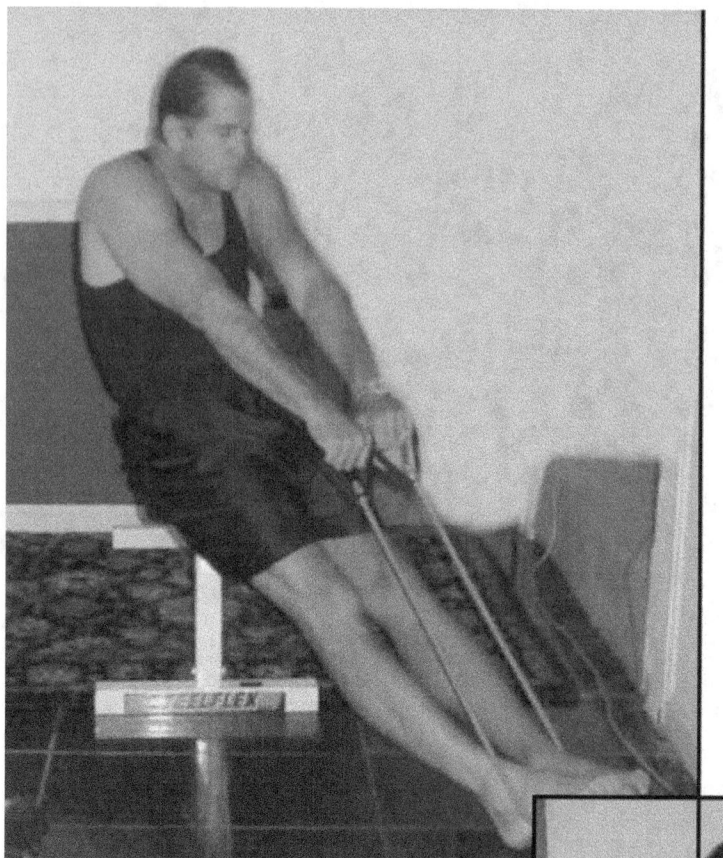

Here we work the lats holding the tube with the feet and the legs locked out in front of the body, lean slightly forward, and then we pull back with the arms

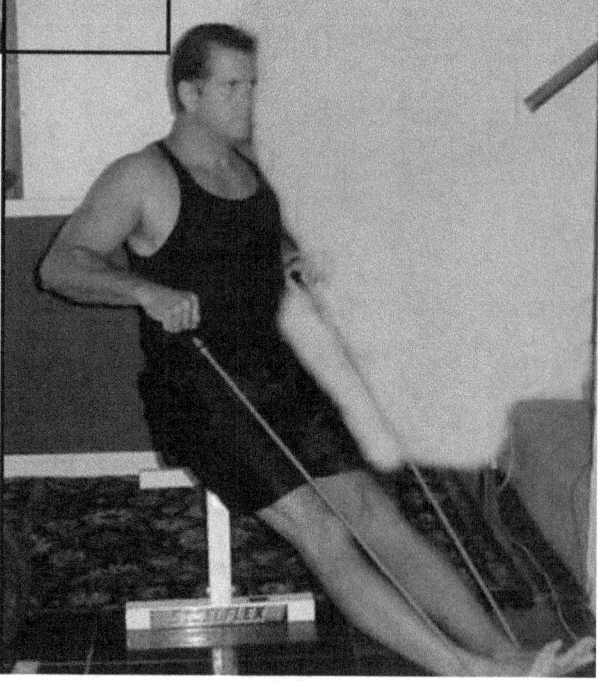

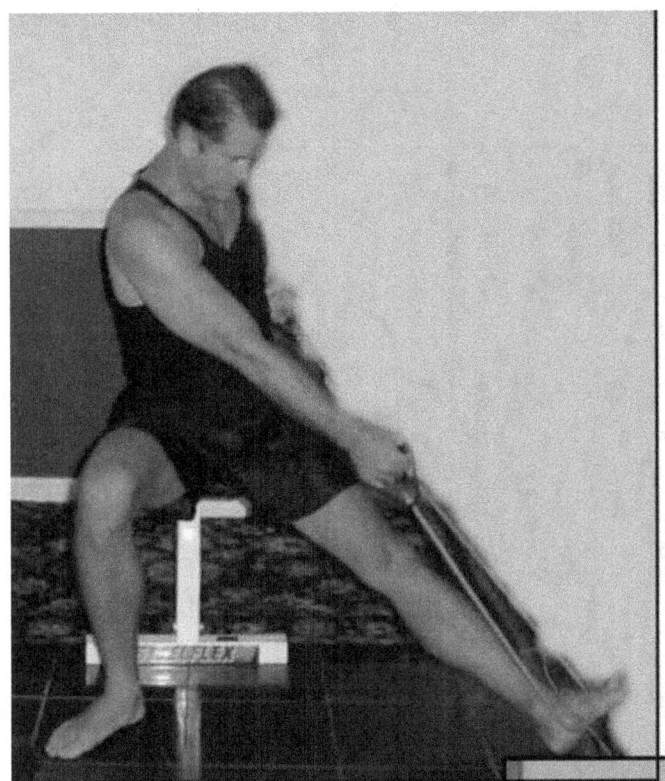

Here we work the lats extending the leg forward and holding the tube with the foot, then pulling back with one arm.

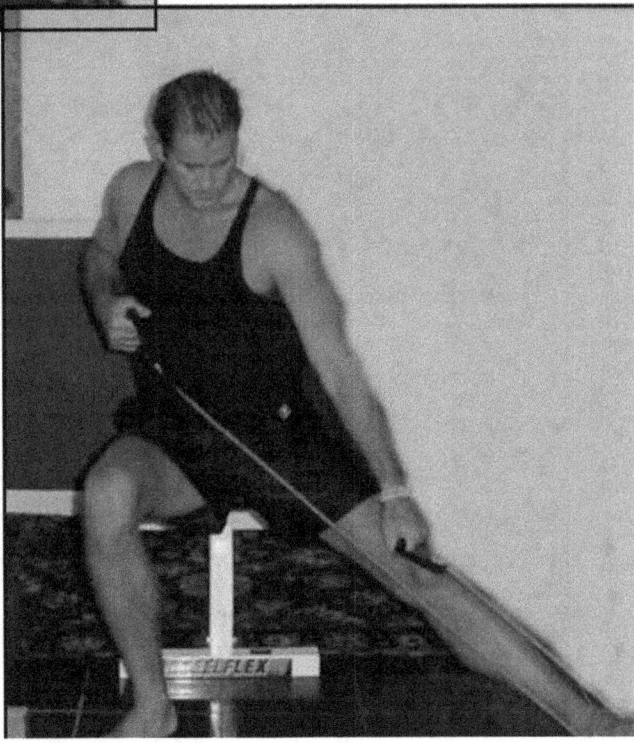

Here we work the
lats leaning forward
holding the tube
with both feet,

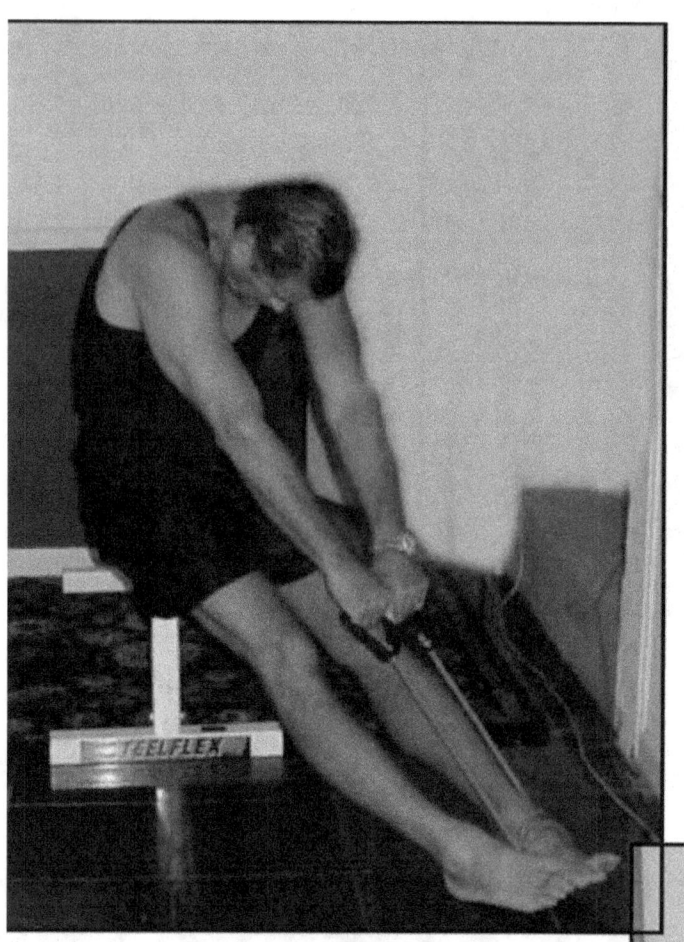

Here we work the
lats leaning
forward holding
the tube with both
feet, leaning
backwards and
pulling the arms to
the side.

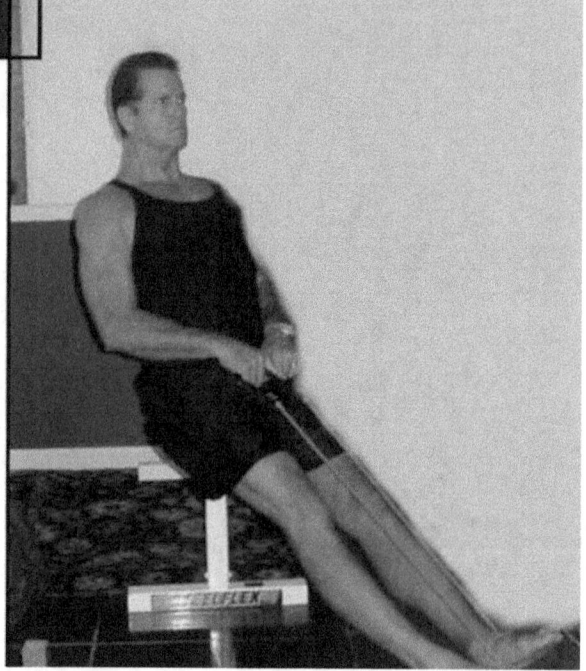